Preparing for Birth and Parenthood

Preparing for Birth and Parenthood

Awareness training and teaching manual for childbirth professionals

Gerlinde M. Wilberg

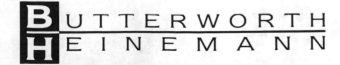

Butterworth-Heinemann Ltd
Linacre House, Jordan Hill, Oxford OX2 8DP

 PART OF REED INTERNATIONAL BOOKS

OXFORD   LONDON   BOSTON
MUNICH   NEW DELHI   SINGAPORE   SYDNEY
TOKYO   TORONTO   WELLINGTON

First published 1992

British Library Cataloguing in Publication Data
A catalogue record for this book is available from the British Library

Library of Congress Cataloguing in Publication Data
A catalogue record for this book is available from the Library of Congress

ISBN 0 7506 0046 2

Printed and bound in Great Britain by
Courier International Limited, East Kilbride

Contents

Part 2 *Physiological Aspects of Antenatal Preparation*

Introduction

Why I wrote this book?

There are plenty of books about natural birth, giving information about different approaches to antenatal preparation and (to) helping women during labour, not to mention the published debates on technological and 'alternative' styles of labour management.

Nevertheless it seems that the entire literature has concentrated exclusively on the 'how?' 'where?' and 'what?' questions:

- HOW would an 'ideal' labour proceed?
- WHERE should it take place?
- WHAT should the parents-to-be know?

'Who?' questions tend to be forgotten:

- WHO are the teachers, and the taught?
- WHO are we, the childbirth professionals and educators?
- WHO are the parents?
- WHO is the unborn child: is he or she indeed recognised as a 'who'?

The formula presented by so many books amounts to the following:

Parents, approaching the unborn child and their own bodies with love and sensitivity	plus	A smooth, natural birth (preferably at home) without interventions
	equals	A contented, happy baby and a successful parent-child relations'

But a child, a newborn human being, is not a sum total of such factors. Good births can no more be *manufactured* than contented babies.

The newborn are stubborn individualists. Some despite dramatic pregnancies and births, go on to lead peaceful, contented lives. Others, despite the most natural and harmonious of introductions to the world, scream in despair against it.

To transmit this understanding:

- that the newborn child brings its own understanding, experience and personality, which may or may not match ours?
- that we can grant this to the newborn and accept our individuality

. . . this is what antenatal teaching means to me in its essence.

> Wanting a child means being prepared to accept a totally new person into our homes and lives, and being prepared to live with this person for the next twenty or so years.

I think that even so-called 'human' labour management needs to reorient itself to the recognition of the baby as an individual.

Not all babies wish to be instantly put to the breast, bathed or carried around anymore than all of them would wish to lie quietly in a warm cot.

Who is this unborn person? How does he or she wish to be born into the world and to be borne within the world?

Finding the right bearing towards the new person requires a basic attitude of openness and receptivity.

It also depends on the parents and who *they* are. What sort of birth will best suit their circumstances, background and needs?

I find it disturbing to see old patterns reappearing in the guise of the new, with one dogma replacing another. Birth within an 'alternative' ward might be 'better' than in a traditional hospital but the same uniformity rules: instead of sterile-robe-and-episiotomy we have naked-squat-and-primal-scream.

Dependence on epidural anaesthetics and heart monitors is replaced by dependence on homeopathy or warm baths.

It scarcely needs saying that neither approach will be right for all women.

And who are we ourselves; the professional birth attendants, doctors, midwives, or antenatal teachers?

What knowledge, experience, expectations, basic attitude and feelings do we bring to bear?

Only by affirming our own individuality instead of wearing the mask of a Lamaze, Kitzinger, Leboyer or Odent can we 'respond' to the individuality of the parents-to-be and the child-to-be.

By 'responsibility' I mean this ability to respond sensitively, ably, to ourselves and the people in our environment.

It is my hope that this handbook will contribute to promoting your human and professional response-ability, in exactly this sense.

What does 'natural birth' mean?

For most of us it means being able to give birth, as women have done for thousands of years and still do in some cultures, without medical help or intervention and surrounded by women who have given birth themselves.

What natural birth should imply is something that comes naturally to us as individuals in the context of our own culture and background. Why should a woman who is used to taking an aspirin for every head - or toothache, not naturally want a pain-killer during labour?

Why should a woman who finds squatting uncomfortable or is embarrassed to go on all fours, not deliver in a lying position, when this is what relaxes her most and enables her to open herself to the experience.

On the other hand we know of the side-effects, not only of medications but also of the horizontal position.

So what is the solution?

In the course of pregnancy most women begin to take their bodies more seriously. They are more careful about taking medicines, and more sensitive to their own body signals: for example their eating and sleeping urges.

This is in itself a natural development, and one which prepares them for childbirth.

I like to compare giving birth to climbing a mountain or going on a marathon. If a woman gives herself over to the birth process and is in tune with her body it won't be an experience of unbearable pain but one which she finds both strenuous and satisfying, as with the long-distance runner.

For the runner too, it is important to breathe properly: no more and no less than the body demands. Only if he exerts unnecessary effort or loses touch with his body will the pain become a spur which works against him and tempts him to give up.

Interesting too that the word 'unbearable' comes from 'to bear' which means 'to give birth'. It is not that childbirth can only be experienced as pain but the other way round. Maybe with every pain we experience, our body wants to give birth metaphorically, wants to express something.

For example when running a marathon or climbing a mountain.
Yet these are clearly not 'everywoman's' thing.
And neither is *birthing*.

Some love it. Some hate it. Some want to go in for it but then within the first few hundred metres decide to take the cable car or the bus after all (in the form of an epidural anaesthetic, for example).

Others are clear in advance that mountain climbing is not to their taste and that they would rather be driven to a peaceful lake.

The fact that she hasn't reached the peak by her own efforts doesn't mean that the woman who takes the cable car cannot enjoy a 'peak experience' of bracing fresh air and an impressive 'view from the top' of her experience.

The question remains, however, what value we allot to the path and the process of scaling the heights. This is where choice rests with the individual woman and the pregnant couple. They must decide what sort of birth they want.

What is unfortunate is that nowadays this free choice is complicated and distorted by a large number of unnecessary and damaging interventions.

Giving birth is in itself a natural process like breathing or digestion. Our body is normally quite capable of handling these processes by itself. Which doctor would find it necessary to monitor normal occurrences of breathing and digestion or a normal circulation of the blood, let alone deliberately tamper with them, speed them up or slow them down.

The body would certainly react to such tampering as to any threat to its own natural mechanisms and integrity, with symptoms and so-called 'complications'.

And yet how frequent are these artificial complications of the birth process in obstetric care.

Medical intervention may indeed be necessary when natural breathing, circulation or birth processes are not running normally.

But how often are these disturbances to natural processes not themselves induced by unnatural beliefs and interventions or the result of an unnatural way of living?

This is why movement, breath and nutritional education, and antenatal education as such, are called for.

Are childbirth preparation and 'natural' birth a contradiction in terms?

"Holding in feelings to maintain self-composure is an unhealthy way to try to be brave. It takes more courage to be who we are, particularly when surrounded by disapproval from medical experts who think they know more about us than we know about ourselves."

Elizabeth Noble

If, despite being confronted with disapproval or interventions, a labouring woman wishes to be in charge of her own unique birthing experience, then she needs to be prepared for it not only physiologically but also emotionally. Conversely, a woman who can be herself and at the same time place total trust in her birth assistants actually needs no special preparation.

In the present climate, childbirth preparation is usually called for.

Normally a pregnant woman has two choices:

- She can hand control over to her birth attendants or she can control herself with learned relaxation and breathing techniques.

On the other hand, if she wishes to dispense with controls, and, despite an unfavourable environment, really opens up to her own process, then she needs another type of preparation. Not techniques and rules, but self-knowledge and self-awareness.

- Knowledge of her own body signals and an instinctive ability to go with them (i.e. a tested and embodied trust, achieved not just through auto-suggestion of the 'My body can give birth' type, but through the experience of exercises and simulated stress).

- Understanding of her own needs and defence mechanisms in the face of stress, disappointment, fear and pain. (Not drilled reaction-tactics but understanding of her own limitations and awareness of the choices available to her in behaviour and response.)

For a woman labouring in adverse circumstances which are all too often the rule, it is essential to be properly aware of her own feelings and body needs, to trust and follow them.

And that must be practised.

Yet if the birth happens in optimal conditions and the woman has a lot of emotional and physical self-confidence she will need no antenatal teaching. Women are able to give birth.

The importance of antenatal teaching is relative.

"Doesn't the female body who knows how to grow a body also know how to birth it?" Elizabeth Noble

If doctors and midwives would treat pregnant women and partners as mature, responsible adults . . ..

If, during check-ups they would attune to and respect the individuality of each woman . . ..

If they would encourage a woman, at each session, to take note of her own body messages – it only requires one well-directed question and time granted to hearken to the answer . . ..

If women and men could trust the birth assistants not to intervene without explanation and good grounds . . . . .

then we would not need 'childbirth preparation'.

If a woman's physical intuition is not undermined but strengthened and the professionals don't meddle unnecessarily, *then 'natural birth' can happen of its own accord*. It can come about naturally.

We, the professionals, must take our own role into consideration. Are we prepared to make ourselves superfluous?

What are we trying to pass on in antenatal teaching?

"Thanks doctor. I wouldn't've managed it without you" used to be the saying. Likewise today one hears people saying "Without my ante-natal teacher I wouldn't've managed. The course taught me exactly what to do and it worked!"

This sort of result could be based on a misinterpretation of the true aim of ante-natal teaching, which is neither to transmit scientific information nor to pass on behaviouristic techniques of breathing and relaxation. It is much more a question of strengthening the confidence of women in their own bodies and in their own authority.

This means:

– My body can bear my child.
– My body knows what it needs.
– I can listen to my body and respond to its signals.
– I know how my body likes to relax itself.
– I know what type of breathing suits my body.
– I am at one with the baby inside me.

If women are given the opportunity to learn this sort of self-confidence in antenatal classes and to share this with their partners, one would expect the following reaction after birth:

"I managed it. My body worked wonderfully. I've never felt so whole before. I've never felt so close to my partner".

What a contrast to the woman who longs nervously and helplessly for the doctor to deliver her, or the woman who, though happy with the way her body functioned, reaps no fulfilment from the experience.

It is certainly not easy for an antenatal teacher to make the change from a course based on psycho-prophylaxis to one based on self-awareness.

– Firstly she must trust her own body and take pleasure in it, otherwise she cannot pass on this self-confidence.

– Secondly she cannot see her own role simply as a dispenser of knowledge (of which she will always possess more than her course participants . . . hence her authority).

– Thirdly, she should not work from the belief that intensive exercise and practice are preconditions for a good labour.

So long as the teacher believes that birth is a complicated business that requires a lot of planning and exercising she will not be preparing women for natural birth.

In the last analysis the quality of an antenatal teacher is not a matter of how much knowledge, or even experience she possesses, but of the degree to which she knows, lives and loves herself as a whole person.

Those who work with, other human beings should know themselves, their own values, motivations and feelings. They must themselves be open and prepared for change if their aim is to reach other people.

Above all else, an antenatal teacher should enjoy working with pregnant women and their partners. If it isn't fun, don't do it.

What type of childbirth preparation is the most 'natural'?

The question behind all the approaches, techniques and exercises for childbirth preparation is whether they don't in fact alienate women from themselves.

Every attempt to influence the behaviour of a labouring woman, no matter how well meant, is an intervention in the natural process.

Medical-technological intervention is often applied unnecessarily and with damaging effect, yet how often do its well-meaning critics end up offering new and alternative interventions, themselves raised to the level of dogma and rule.

It is not a question of certain methods being better than others but of the fact that there are no methods of childbirth preparation or assistance that can suit so individual an experience as birth in every case.

Why then are new methods constantly thought up, and taken up, for something that actually needs no method at all?

Every method has its principles and rules which imply somehow that the birth process is predictable and controllable, and it is this element of control that attracts not only the childbirth professionals but also pregnant women and their partners themselves.

Antenatal teaching often remains stuck at the level of making the birth process intellectually understandable only, whilst at the same time criticising current birthing procedures and methods.

The over-stressing of factual knowledge goes hand in hand with training in techniques of control, for example in dealing with contractions.

Hidden standards are set for a 'natural' birth which promote a new dependency and strip parents of whatever self-confidence they had.

The antenatal teacher becomes the expert, leaving parents in the role of passive consumers. More and better rules to follow are supplied. Fine, there's nothing wrong with improving the rules, but what if they don't suit the individuals concerned?

Childbirth preparation should, in the first place, encourage parents to find out and decide for themselves what they want; what sort of birth and what sort of assistance in birth. It should furthermore make them better able to understand their own physical and psychological changes, awakening in them the readiness and openness to find their own individual way through the birth experience.

Why is the self-awareness dimension so important?

How a birth turns out (whether, for example complications or intense pains occur) depends on the psychological background of the labouring woman. And, many would also say, on her physical constitution, her genetic background, and her birth environment. But these too, are influenced by the psychological factor.

What is the psychological background to a birth?

- The experience of one's own birth (including what one was told about it).
- The experience of one's own mother and the parental home.
- The experience of socialisation (cultural influences).

These experiences affect our basic attitudes to birth:

- Our attitude to nutrition, and how we relate to our own bodies.
- Our attitude to mother- and fatherhood, whether we want children, etc.
- Our attitude to sexuality, femininity and masculinity in ourselves.
- Our attitude to orthodox medicine, whether we are critical, informed, able to express our wishes, etc.
- Our orientation to life, positive or negative; whether we need drama, prefer comedy, fear boredom, etc.

These basic attitudes in turn leave their mark on our life script:

- Our present life with or without a partner.
- Our physical health and fitness.
- Our choice of hospital/midwife/birth style.

I believe it is important to accept and take responsibility for our own lives and for what happens to us, instead of blaming external factors: a bad birth environment, poor constitution, fate, etc.

We cannot reverse the past but we can check out and change the beliefs that resulted from it, and thus rewrite our life script.

How you can use this book

This book is for all who come into contact professionally with pregnant or labouring women.

The first part contains guided reflections, questions and meditations on themes of critical relevance to childbirth preparation.

The units are there for you to work through in your own time over the coming months or years. Choose the theme that you feel most relevant to *you* at any given time.

Have pen, paper or a cassette recorder to hand. If you can, arrange time for sessions with someone prepared to listen to the reflections inspired by the theme.

Choose the way of working (writing, recording, or arranging time with a listener) that you feel most comfortable with. If you are working with a recorder or listener, try the techniques: 'Rosary' and 'Mutual questioning' (see p.173).

A good listener should accept and respect you even when you express negative feelings. He or she should be capable of understanding and empathy, but on the other hand the listeners should not be so directly or personally involved with the themes themselves as to influence your train of thought by their own reactions. They must be capable of silence.

Try to find someone who probably knows less about psychology than you do. This way, if they are tempted to interpret your utterances, you will find it easier to ignore such interpretations. You can remind your listener that you are only thinking aloud and that the purpose of this is to work things through yourself.

If you prefer to put your thoughts down on paper, choose a pen that writes fluidly, without worrying about legibility, grammar or punctuation.

No-one else should read it except you.

You are talking to yourself in writing.

Try to write in a continuous stream, without second thoughts or corrections.

Write everything that comes to you, even if its relevance is not obvious.

If you find yourself slowing down or getting stuck, copy the questions out again, in order to keep on writing. A continuous flow of script or of speech has a hypnotic effect and will take you further than holding back or pausing for thought.

If writing doesn't suit you and you can't find a good listener it's a good idea to record your thoughts aloud on tape. Not necessarily in order to play them back, but simply as a stimulus to your own flow of speech.

Work section by section within each unit.

Answer each question as soon as you read it.

Reading to the end of each unit first will most likely prejudice your answers. It will also mean that you cannot *compare* the answers you gave to those you might feel you would have wanted to give when you come to the end of the unit. This can be a source of discovery.

Remember that this is no test, with 'right' or 'wrong' answers, but a resource to help you find *your* answers.

In the second and third parts of the book you will find a collection of exercises relating to different aspects of childbirth preparation. These are also prefaced with guided reflections and personal questions to consider. Work through these as with Part 1. The exercises themselves are intended as models only, to be used, or altered for use, as required.

Some of the information, reflections or attitudes presented in this book will appear as prescriptive or bold. You are invited to question any statement or exercise.

What I write is not meant as an absolute truth to be followed but rather as a challenge for you to find your own belief or the stance you would like to take on any particular issue.

PART 1 Guided Reflections on the Issues and Attitudes Influencing Childbirth Preparation

Many of us carry a burden of problems, feelings and inner conflicts; we drag them around with us like a heavy suitcase. Some of us know exactly what the suitcase contains; monthly, weekly or daily we sort through and examine its contents, only to carefully pack them in again and continue carrying them around, complainingly, proudly, or silently. Others of us have no idea what we are carrying — an assortment of memories and experiences and grievances from the near or distant past. And we do not want to look into our suitcase at all. Still, we carry it with us, like a collection of old clothes that will never be worn again but are never put away. Others of us, still, realizing suddenly that we do not need this burden, simply put our suitcases down and walk away. Yet some of us lighten our load bit by bit, throwing away the contents of the suitcase piece by piece, taking one last look and keeping only what we want and need.

1 Individuality – accepting yourself

If our goal is to help pregnant women and their partners to accept their own individuality, then we, too, must accept our individuality. Accepting ourselves means:

- Getting to know ourselves
- Becoming more conscious of ourselves
- Respecting our own body language, including symptoms
- Allowing ourselves to feel our feelings
- Living and expressing our own multiplicity and contradictory feelings.

There are two distinct levels on which we can accept ourselves. Choose for yourself the one that is right for you.

EXAMPLES

- Can you accept that though usually aware of your own body signals, you tend not to respect them?
  Can you accept your body signals to the extent of actually respecting and heeding them?
- Can you accept that you tend to either hide your strengths or to show them off?
  Can you accept your strengths to such a degree that you need to neither hide nor show them off?
- Can you accept that you tend to either fight your own weaknesses or to minimize them?
  Can you accept your weaknesses without either fighting or minimizing them?
- Can you accept that you either use sarcasm in asserting yourself or abandon your rights out of pity for the other person?

Can you accept your own rights so fully that you can act on them without sarcasm or pity?

It is important to realize that we all have a choice: we need neither reach the second level nor stay with the first. But we need to let ourselves know where we stand, and to accept our limitations. Self-awareness and self-confidence grow from this.

2 Strengths and weaknesses

Once upon a time, there was a child who kept being annoyed by a little devil. The devil pinched him, scratched him, and whispered evil thoughts in his ear. The child tried to push the devil away, saying 'Go away! I don't like you!' But the little devil sneaked secretly back.

The more the child tried to fend the devil off, the more cunning the devil became. He came back more and more often, sneaking up from behind when the child wasn't thinking of him. Wherever the child went the devil followed.

Eventually the child could think of or do nothing else than try to break free from the devil.

Then he had an idea. He took the devil firmly in his arms, cuddled and stroked him like a teddy bear and said: 'Now you belong to me. You can stay with me and I won't try to send you away again.' And with this the devil started to feel quite at ease. That was after all, what he had wanted all the time . . . to be acknowledged and accepted! The child hugged him closely and said: 'I like you. You're mine.'

Instead of being naughty the devil became lovable. He enjoyed living with the child and the child enjoyed living with him. They had fun together.

Now that the little devil didn't disturb him any more the child finally had time for all his other games, and didn't need to fight the devil all day. The devil even helped him to build his big tower of blocks, instead of always knocking them down.

When asked to reflect on their strengths and weaknesses, participants in training often exclaim how difficult they find praising or criticizing themselves.

However, if we can learn to own and accept ourselves with all our weaknesses and strengths then, as in the opening story, we will no longer be trapped. It's when we try to ignore our weaknesses or strengths, try to deny or avoid them, that they unbalance our lives, our work and our relationships. If, on the other hand, we can accept them we can not only take them in hand but also use them creatively.

Let us examine our strengths and weaknesses more closely.

REFLECTIONS   **1** Make a list of all your weaknesses that come to mind. Now look through your list:
- which of these weaknesses can you accept? (OK, that's how I am, and that's how I want to be . . .)
- which of the weaknesses do you feel are destructive, or are not an integral part of you?

2 Write down a list of all your strengths. Now look at the list:
- which strengths do you use and when?
  are there strengths that you show only in particular situations, with particular people? If so, why?
- which strengths are dormant in you? What do you need in order to bring them out?

Every weakness can, at the same time, be a strength. Similarly each strength can also be a weakness. A strength can easily turn into a weakness if you are not aware of it, or use it unthinkingly.

EXAMPLE

One of my strengths is being intuitive. But if I express it unthinkingly it can also come out as prejudice. I cannot use my strength blindly; I have to use it consciously. I need to check it out – is it really intuition or are there other feelings at work?

3 Think of examples of your own strengths. What sort of weaknesses could these turn into? What do you have to watch out for?

But how can a weakness turn into a strength?

EXAMPLE

Alice runs evening classes. She is a fairly reserved person and doesn't easily let people get close. Alice clearly has a weakness in a job that brings her constantly into close contact with others. Yet by acknowledging and embodying this weakness more consciously it can become a strength allowing her to establish boundaries and stay within them. A positive aspect of this for Alice is that it allows her to guard her own interests. A positive aspect for the participants is that it strengthens their independence.

But weakness has to be acknowledged fully in order to make it work this way. If we struggle against our own feelings in order to overcome them, and, as in Alice's case, don't allow ourselves any distance from the participants, we will sooner or later end up exhausted. Just knowing about a weakness isn't enough. It has to be accepted and lived. That way it becomes a strength.

Some other thoughts:
- – do I really need my weakness in order to live out my strengths?
- – why do I cling to my weaknesses?
- – why do I believe that giving up my weaknesses means giving up my strengths?

It does not need to be so. There are other ways of showing strengths, that do not rely on weaknesses. Let us clarify the last example, and in so doing show how the ability to establish boundaries can be carried through.

A teacher brings an evening class to an end at exactly 10.00pm because she is afraid that if she extends the session it won't just be a matter of five minutes extra.

> 'One member of my class has tears in her eyes. If we do carry on for a while she'll begin to cry . . . and most likely phone me tomorrow morning just as I'm getting the children ready for school . . . so the sooner we finish the better!'

She needs to use the time limit to protect herself.

Another teacher brings the class to an end at exactly 10.00pm because she knows that although there is a lot that remains to be said, they can't deal with everything in one night. The class members need time to digest things and so does she.

> 'One of them has tears in her eyes. I ask her at the door if she would like a chance to talk about it. If she says yes I tell her to phone me at an agreed time in the morning.'

This teacher has learned to protect her own interests.

4 Think of alternative ways of expressing your strengths which don't rely on the corresponding weaknesses. Can you imagine having the strengths without the weaknesses? Can you accept that as you are now, you may need the weaknesses?

5 Make a list of qualities that you know might be interpreted in a variety of ways by different people or groups of people (aggressiveness, self-sacrifice, childishness, naivety). Then look at the list and mark those which you clearly think represent either weaknesses or strengths
- – how do you feel about qualities which you understand as strengths but which others see as weaknesses? Can you stand by them?
- – how do you feel about qualities which you interpret as weaknesses but which others regard as strengths? Can you accept them?
- – think about those qualities which you find difficult to classify. Can you see anything they have in common?
- – are there a few or many of these ambiguous qualities? How do you feel about this? Can you accept them?

6 Draw a diagram of the weaknesses and strengths important in your work with pregnant women and parents-to-be.

Draw connecting lines and arrows. See which qualities influence or give rise to each other. Talk or write about the points you need to watch for in applying or exploiting your strengths and weaknesses. Talk or write about the concrete changes you can make in your work so as to fully exploit, balance, or hold in-check the relevant strengths and weaknesses

EXAMPLE

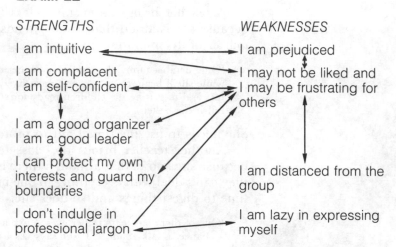

STRENGTHS

I am intuitive

I am complacent

I am self-confident

I am a good organizer
I am a good leader

I can protect my own
interests and guard my
boundaries

I don't indulge in
professional jargon

WEAKNESSES

I am prejudiced

I may not be liked and
I may be frustrating for
others

I am distanced from the
group

I am lazy in expressing
myself

3 One's own experience of birth

'One's own experience of birth' does not just mean one's own birth or the birth of one's children, but all births that one has experienced or taken part in.

The broader the range of this experience, the better of course.

- An antenatal teacher who has witnessed three completely different births has a wider range of experience than one who has seen 20 with routine episiotomies and doses of pethidine
- A midwife who has only seen births in which syntometrin was injected will find it difficult to believe that the uterus can contract strongly enough to release the placenta by itself
- A doctor who has delivered hundreds of babies, but only in hospitals, may have difficulty in accepting that women can also deliver safely at home
- An antenatal teacher who has never experienced a well-handled Second Stage may find it difficult to communicate that it is enough to breathe calmly and to push only when the urge is felt.

Although one's personal experience of birth may not have been the main factor influencing our decision to work with pregnant women, it has an undeniable effect on the way we do so, and also on our relations with (other) midwives and doctors.

A midwife who herself had a beautiful pregnancy and a birth free of complications may find it hard to understand the aches and pains and difficulties experienced by other women. Similarly, a doctor who, to be on the safe side, performed a Caesarian in delivering his own wife may find it difficult to be a good assistant at a 'natural birth'. On the other hand, an antenatal teacher who delivered at home, may find it difficult to support fully parents who wish for a hospital birth.

REFLECTIONS   1 Find your own examples of similar situations.

Saying that people 'may find it difficult' does not mean that it is impossible nor that, as a rule, we cannot talk about things we have not directly experienced ourselves. Yet, to make this possible we need to take our personal experience into account and learn to see it as part of a broader picture. Otherwise, what we say to pregnant women and couples will inevitably be tinged with this experience. However theoretically balanced we try to be, it is what they hear 'between the lines' that will influence them most.

The critical points are our personal experiences of:

○ Specific stages of pregnancy and labour
○ Assisting/being present at the birth
○ Hospital/home delivery
○ Pain relief
○ Medical intervention

It is a question of checking out how strongly we are influenced by our own experiences in these areas:

– does our experience match the conventional wisdom?
– what do we really believe?
– are our beliefs based on theory, on personal experience, or the integration of both?

2 Try to find out about your own birth from parents, relatives, older brothers or sisters. Put all the information together and write a report on your own birth, embroidering the details if necessary.

Sticking to the facts (circumstances, timing, complications etc.) write several versions of the report, according to how the birth might have been seen or experienced. Which version do you wish not to have been true? Which do you wish would have been true? Which version sounds most realistic? Can you discover any pointers to your current attitudes to pregnancy and birth? Make a list of your attitudes beginning each sentence with 'Because my birth was like this . . .'.

3 Write a subjective account of the birth of your child/ren as experienced by:

○ You
○ Your partner
○ The baby
○ Your midwife/doctor

Allow yourself to see the birth from as many perspectives as possible.

4 Write different birth reports, for example:

○ The best labour you can imagine or have experienced
○ The worst labour you can imagine or have experienced

5 Make a list of the insights that you have gained from your experience of birth.

EXAMPLE

'Although I was in a lying down position during the first stage I am sure that an upright position would be better for most women'.

6 Write two versions of a birth you have experienced, one positive and one negative. In particular, if there was a labour you experienced negatively, try and reinterpret it in a positive validating way.

This exercise can be particularly useful as a further reflection on our own values. When reading through birth reports try to distinguish between fact and interpretation. Behind many a glowing report quite a few complications may be concealed and, conversely, many subjectively negative reports hide normal labour processes. It is an excellent idea to share such observations with your classes – by reading aloud to them an account of a birth in two versions. This will help them to accept their own birth experience in its own terms, and not prejudice that experience with distorting criteria and interpretation.

Whilst it is a good thing to have high positive expectations for one's labour and for the birth event, it is unhelpful if these expectations are so fixed that any variation or unpredictability is seen automatically as negative. There is a difference between genuine 'positive thinking' and the sort of thinking that imposes restrictive requirements on events as *conditions* for a positive experience.

EXAMPLE

A woman can be very clear in herself that the screams she is uttering are not screams of pleasure or relief but of pain or anger. She doesn't need to persuade herself that she is not feeling any pain or fury, but nor does she need to interpret her feelings and their expression negatively. She can allow herself to feel disappointed at having such ugly feelings or can pride herself on having granted these feelings their own powerful voice.

There should be no pressure in classes towards the attitude that 'whatever happens in labour I have to experience it positively'. The point is rather to raise the couples' awareness of how certain interpretations or false attitudes (like 'screaming is bad' or 'lying down is bad') can themselves influence that experience negatively. This is particularly important if the woman herself is unsure of her own values, attitudes and beliefs, and therefore susceptible to those of her attendants.

EXAMPLE OF A BIRTH REPORT IN TWO VERSIONS

On December 29th I had a dental appointment. Going to the toilet before I left the house I noticed I had a bloody secretion: the first sign . . .

I was so happy and excited knowing it was all about to start today, I couldn't eat a thing all afternoon. Obviously my body had already geared itself up to the coming contractions and didn't want to waste any energy on digestion.

I freaked out. There was an hour's drive ahead of me to the dentist and it was all too much. I was so restless all afternoon I couldn't eat a thing and was worried that I wouldn't have enough energy for the labour.

As evening approached contractions began to come regularly, every seven or eight minutes. They lasted almost a minute, but were mild and easy to breathe through.

I felt calm and relaxed, put my 4-year-old son to bed, sang him bedtime songs and took pleasure in the flow of contractions. Everything seemed so meaningful and the timing seemed just right: Jonah would sleep and we would have the night for ourselves.

My nerves had completely given out. Contractions seemed to come for hours at the same frequency. Nothing changed . . . as if it could go on like this all night . . . and I hadn't slept all day. Not to mention having to put Jonah to bed. It was an effort to control myself.

At about 10.00pm I phoned the midwife to let her know what was happening. The contractions were still mild and the frequency hadn't changed. In the intervals we played a version of noughts and crosses. Each game was just long enough to fill the pauses between contractions.

I was so full of energy, joy and lightness I surprised even myself! I'd never have thought that I could be playing games during first stage; at the last birth everything had been so serious and intense. The midwife wanted to come immediately but I told her that Peter and I wanted to savour the atmosphere of this time together alone for a while.

I was restless not knowing if these contractions were the real thing or not. If the frequency didn't change shouldn't they at least increase in intensity? How long would this go on for? The midwife wanted to come immediately but I told her I wasn't sure if labour had really begun. Everything seemed wrong. I played noughts and crosses in the intervals between contractions. I was so worked up I didn't know what else to do.

At about 11.00pm the midwife came. Her internal examination showed that I was already 4–5 cm dilated. Soon after the contractions grew more intense and began to come every four minutes.

Great! I'd never have believed that such mild contractions could bring about so much dilation. I hadn't reckoned on such an easy first stage, and now I found myself overjoyed, laughing after each contraction and amazed at their strength.

Horrors! Already so dilated – it's really going to happen tonight! Soon they'll be getting even more intense and painful. I was so worked up I laughed nervously after each contraction instead of concentrating calmly.

I walked around or leaned forwards over the sofa or kitchen cupboard. I drank raspberry leaf tea.

I felt so good and full of energy. The sofa became my 'point of power'. I could really sense how the energy streamed through me, yet between contractions I could move freely, and wandered to and fro between bedroom, kitchen and living room. I didn't need to cling to any one position. The force was with me.

Why was I so restless, constantly changing my position and never able to stay with it? I went from one room to another needing to lean forwards on a support when contractions came. Why couldn't I just find one position to relax in? It was all so different from my expectations.

From midnight on, intense back pains accompanied each contraction; so much so I thought my back would burst.

I knew exactly what I needed for each contraction: sometimes to rotate my pelvis, sometimes just Peter's warm hand on a point near my coccyx, sometimes firm pressure. I would tell Peter what I wanted and he reacted wonderfully despite my sometimes rough commands: 'Leave it!' 'No, further down!' 'Firmer!' 'No, no, Leave it!' It was a unique experience, responding second by second to my body's exact needs.

I was totally dominated by the back pains. Nothing seemed to help even though we tried everything: pelvic rotations, warmth, pressure. They all seemed to help for a few seconds but then the pains were back with full force. I was very rough with Peter and kept on ordering him about. Where were the loving looks and kisses that we were supposed to be enjoying?

The backbreaking pains changed. Now, each contraction put pressure on the anus; a sign of second stage. We moved into position in the bedroom. Mirror between my legs I leant on/hung from Peter's shoulders. The downward pressure of the contractions was incredible. Our midwife knelt behind me ready to catch the baby. No internal examination to make sure. She relied on what I sensed.

There was a good atmosphere of mutual trust. Being in a half squatting position she couldn't hear the baby's heartbeat, and yet knowing I wanted to stay this way she didn't insist once that I lie down between contractions for her to listen in. There was a tremendous, timeless energy in the room. I babbled in nonsense language during each contraction – it was the only way for me to keep breathing. And in each interval I hung relaxed and exhausted

The contractions were incredibly painful. Jonah's second stage had been easy by comparison. I was totally overwhelmed, dependent on one position and on Peter. Yet when his trousers got bloodstained I told him to go and soak them in cold water. Why am I still bothered with things like that? I am too detached on the one hand and totally dependent on the other – for when the next contraction came, and Peter was still out of from Peter's arms. He was a steady tower throughout this hour. I could completely let go. It was a total physical experience and yet I was still mentally alert. In fact I had to smile at myself inwardly for still being concerned at bloodstains on Peter's trousers and making appreciative professional observations of our midwife's non-interfering manner.

the room I was absolutely helpless. Having critical thoughts of the midwife too. Shouldn't she insist on an internal examination? Shouldn't she listen to the baby's heartbeat? Yet I feel unable to change my position or even control my breathing. I spout nonsense during each contraction and despise myself for neither being in control nor surrendering completely.

Slowly the head moved further down. A yellow-white amniotic sac hangs out of my vagina. I feel no urge to push.

I could give in to the contractions completely now. Trusting in the baby pushing down, relaxing fully in Peter's arms and opening myself to what is happening. Giving birth is tremendous, unique, wonderful.

Why do I feel no urge to push? Why is everything going so slowly? How long can I hold out? Is this normal? Is the baby all right? Why isn't the midwife doing anything? When will it finally be over?

The midwife broke the waters and suddenly I felt the urge to push. I lay back on the bed so that the midwife could see and take care of my perineum, breathed, and pressed the head and shoulders out. It was a terrible exertion, and painful as hell. I felt as if everything in me was tearing. As the head emerged I let out a loud cry.

A primal scream! With this birth I've really explored the limits of my physical being and fulfilled them. What a wonder, what a gift for us women to experience. I felt blessed and was euphoric for weeks after.

It was terrible! It wasn't my idea of second stage. No orgasmic breathing, no opening like a flower. Instead this awful scream. I felt I'd let myself down, failed the test of my own womanhood. Was depressed for days and weeks after.

This example illustrates that the birth process is not a product of external circumstances (the hospital, the midwives, which doctors on duty etc.) or of inner biological circumstances (size and position of the baby, hormone balance, strength of contractions etc.). Rather, it is our attitudes, beliefs and interpretations which influence not only our experience of birth but the actual course of the labour. On the one hand (right column) the woman had no concrete expectations for her labour: she was ready for anything, and had trust in herself, her partner, and her midwife. On the other hand (left column) the woman had concrete expectations: she wanted a gentle 'picture-book' birth, and to prove herself and her femininity with this. She was uncertain of herself, her partner, and her midwife. Whether we feel essentially positive or negative influences our relationship to our birth attendants and to our own hormonal balance which in turn affect the process of labour.

4 Motivation

We all have many reasons for wanting to work with pregnant women and their partners. But motivation has many layers: some obvious, some concealed; some which fit together perfectly, some which appear to be ill-matched. Whatever our motivation, you can be sure that it finds expression in the way we work. It is valuable, therefore, to reflect on ourselves: to discover which of our motivations really fire us, which of them act as brakes, and which of them are double-edged.

What follows is a relaxation exercise leading to a guided recollection to help you explore your own motivation. Ask someone to read it aloud to you (it will take about 20 minutes) making sure that they do so slowly and with suitable pauses.

Exercise

RELAXATION

Close your eyes.

Allow your body to relax and become soft.

Don't force anything, just let your body slowly melt into any position it wants.

Give it time. Let it happen gradually . . .

Be aware of all your sensations.

Let yourself know what your body wants and needs.

Respond to those you can respond to (loosening clothes or shifting position).

Acknowledge that there are some you can't respond to just yet but can still listen too.

Allow each breath to enter and leave you freely.

If this isn't immediately possible, then allow a sigh with each outbreath – not forced, but just enough to let go, to release your breath, to release your tension.

(And if you find yourself sighing in pressured, high tones let deeper tones come through – uuuuu aaaaa ooooo . . .)

Give yourself over to the breathing.

Let it move you.

Become aware of which parts of your body move when you breathe; ribcage, belly . . . let the breath movements extend wider and further, but don't force anything; just observe and be breathed.

And now, if you are comfortable, just remain sitting or lying.

Rest in yourself for a few minutes.

And if you are not totally comfortable, allow yourself to stretch and yawn a bit till you are.

And come to rest in yourself.

Feel yourself becoming softer and softer . . .

GUIDED RECOLLECTION: MOTIVATION

And now be prepared to go on a small journey into your past.

You don't need to force anything.

Just let your thoughts wander, and let them be guided with a few suggestions.

Only observe what wells up before your inner eye.

Trust whatever thoughts and pictures come up.

Let's begin with the present.

Allow a picture to emerge of this time and space, this room and yourself within it, the way you are lying or sitting.

Acknowledge how you see yourself and how you feel.

Then let the picture melt away.

Wander further back in your thoughts to the point at which you first settled down in this room.

How did you feel then? What thoughts and pictures do you have of this point in time?

Now go slowly back through the day, and think of all the things you have done.

How did you feel when you got up this morning?

Take note of all the memories and feelings that arise.

Don't force anything, just observe them like a film.

Now wander further back through last week.

Let small, forgotten incidents return to you.

Moments in which you were totally yourself.

Moments in which you were very different from how you are now.

See what comes to you and wander further and further back through the week.

Don't hang on to any thoughts.

Let pictures emerge and then melt away.

Don't try and produce memories.

Just see what emerges of itself.

Everything is of equal value. You don't need to choose, but just follow your thoughts wherever they go.

Now wander further back through recent weeks, months and years and let memories rise up.

Which situations and encounters stimulated your desire to work in this field of childbirth?

If you recall a situation, acknowledge it, observe it, recognize other people involved and let yourself feel again what you were feeling then.

Let the memories come alive: the circumstances, the people, the feelings.

And give yourself time.

Just observe what comes up.

Perhaps it is situations that seem irrelevant, but acknowledge them for what they might offer.

Now allow yourself to recall that situation or encounter which first led you in the direction of your present work in the birth field, that planted the seeds of this work.

Simply see what comes up.

Acknowledge everything without being selective.

Let memories form and disappear, feelings too, however irrational they may seem.

Don't judge, just allow and acknowledge.

Give yourself time to recall the various situations and encounters until you have the feeling that that was it! That's where it started!

Give yourself time and see what comes up.

> When you feel that you are finished or that you've had enough, yawn and stretch a bit, breathe deeply. Slowly pick up your pen and write down in your own time all the events that rose from your memory.
>
> Don't be selective. Just write them all down.

REFLECTIONS

1 Answer two of the following sets of questions in writing or with a partner:

(a) What *role* does childbirth preparation play in your life?
What role does *childbirth preparation* play in your life?
What role does childbirth preparation play in *your* life?

(b) What would your life be like *without* childbirth preparation?
What would your life be like without *childbirth preparation*?
What would *your* life be like without childbirth preparation?

(c) How *strongly* is your life influenced by childbirth preparation?
How strongly is your life influenced by *childbirth preparation*?
How strongly is *your* life influenced by childbirth preparation?

(d) How does childbirth preparation *alter* your life?
How does *childbirth preparation* alter your life?
How does childbirth preparation alter *your* life?

For 'childbirth preparation' feel free to substitute any term more appropriate to your professional involvement in the birth field e.g. 'your work as a midwife/obstetric nurse/gynaecologist'.

Pair exercise (approx. 10 min.)

If you choose to work with a partner:
Partner A puts each version of the questions in turn to B using the appropriate intonation. If B seems stuck or there seems more that he or she could say the question is repeated. The whole cycle of questions may be repeated as many times as necessary.   (5–7 min.)
A summarizes B's answers.   (2 min.)
B confirms whether or not this summary reflects his or her intended statements.   (1 min.)

The object of the exercise is to become aware that our original motivation is not, by itself, enough to keep us going in our work but that we need constantly to refuel our motivation through reflection.

2 Write, tell a listener, or record on tape the following:
– what fires my motivation?
– what keeps the flame burning?
– what sort of situations or events give me fresh inspiration?

Remember that we neither always *can* nor *wish* to work with total enthusiasm or unlimited energy.

3 Write, tell a listener, or record on tape the following:
  – what inhibits my work sometimes?
  – what situations or events are most inhibiting or draining of motivation?

The main cause of loss of motivation is not getting enough satisfaction from our work. If what we are doing doesn't satisfy any needs of our own how can it motivate us?

4 Write, tell a listener, or record on tape the following:
  – which of your needs does your work in the field of childbirth satisfy? (Write everything that comes to mind, no matter how surprising or tangential it may seem.)
  – which qualities does your work bring out of you? (Spontaneity, authority, calmness, sociability etc.)
  – what does your work with pregnant women and their partners give you? (Power, authority, money, insight etc.)

5 Make a list of your needs. When you can't think of any more rank them in order of importance. Then ask yourself:
  – which needs are the most vital for me to satisfy?
  – which are met and which are not satisfied in my work?
  – where do the ones which remain unsatisfied rank in my original list?
  – are there important needs which are unfulfilled?
  – are there unimportant needs which are fulfilled?
  – or do I feel that my important needs are satisfied?

There is nothing wrong with having our own needs acknowledged. But it is important that we recognize them for ourselves. If we deny our own needs it is still possible to respond to the needs of others, but more often than not our unmet needs create bitterness and frustration which then creeps into our work and tarnishes our relations with others, and influences what we give (or deny) *them*. These considerations are important not just for us but also for the pregnant women themselves. Always bear in mind two key questions:
  – what do *I* need this work for?
  – what do *I* want from my work?

5   Aims of antenatal teaching

What are the aims of an antenatal class? Do they match up to norms and attitudes, and the exercises you offer?

The norms encountered in training courses fall into two categories: the desired norms which reflect the attitudes of the teacher, and what we might call the undesired norms which the teacher may have to face in reality.

EXAMPLES

Desired norms

Couples with a good relationship wanting a home birth or at least a natural birth without medication.

Mothers who will give up work for at least a year, breastfeed for nine months, carry the child round with them etc.

Undesired norms

Individuals with high standards wanting a private consultant but not really interested in natural birth.

Wanting to spend the first days in hospital without rooming in.

Giving up all manner of activities including sports and hobbies in the first months of pregnancy.

Going back to work after a few months.

No breast feeding.

REFLECTIONS

1 Make a list of your own positive and negative norms. You may be surprised to discover some of them. You may wish to review or reconsider others. There may be some you wish to make sure you don't impose on people or bully them into.

It often happens that there are contradictions between the goals we set and the beliefs and norms we bring to bear in realizing them.

Examples of some contradictory objective setting in antenatal classes:

1. Aim

   To enable couples to clarify their own needs and wishes and make their own choices.

   Belief of teacher

   Home birth; no medication; child should sleep in parents' bed; nine months' breastfeeding etc.

   Content of course

   Information about medical interventions, bad nutritional habits, dangers of psychological damage to babies and infants.

   Result

   The couple go away feeling more nervous and insecure. In addition they now feel guilty about not being able to live up to the norms set by the teacher.

2. Aim

   To help women to breathe freely in the way that comes naturally to them according to their own bodies.

   Belief of teacher

   Couples need something tangible to grasp. Lamaze breathing worked with me so . . .

   Content of course

   Strict adherence to the Lamaze method.

   Result

   Insecurity.

3. Aim

   To communicate the message to women that they only need to push in second stage when and as they feel the urge.

   Belief of teacher

   This won't be possible in our local hospitals.

   Content of course

   Information and exercises in line with the aim are bracketed and qualified: 'This would be ideal, and it's a good idea to try it, but . . . '

   Result

   Insecurity.

4. Aim

   Couples should be independent and self-confident in carrying through their own decisions.

   Belief of teacher

   Couples must be offered all available time and energy.

   Content of course

   The teacher is always available for a talk and whenever possible attends the birth.

   Result

   The couples enjoy being mothered but the aim is not realized, and the teacher is overstretched.

2 Make a list of the subject areas you think should be included in an antenatal course, and find matching goals for each element. Alternatively, make a list of goals and then a matching contents list (with exercises if you wish to go further).

PRINCIPLES AND AIMS OF ANTENATAL CLASSES

These are to:

1. Recognize that every course is different, and to respect the nature and needs of each group.
2. Ensure that pregnancy, birth and parenthood reflect the individual needs of the parents and of the child.
3. Encourage trust in one's own body. This is more important than knowledge or physical fitness.
4. Educate on the realities of pregnancy, birth, and life with a child. Beliefs, norms and values are reflected upon here.
5. Transmit the following:
   ○ Trust, sensitivity and responsiveness to one's own body
   ○ Knowledge of what goes on in pregnancy and birth, including medical and antenatal care, hospital routines and assistance during labour etc. (What is normal/helpful/ unnecessary/damaging?)
   ○ Ways of helping oneself (breathing rhythms, herb teas, positions, breastfeeding counselling, support groups etc.)
   ○ One's own rights and the possibilities for making birth easier and more comfortable (self-assertiveness).
6. Offer preparation for parenthood. This is achieved by:
   ○ Reflections on the child in pregnancy
   ○ Reflections on anticipation of family life (integrating parenthood in one's identity)
   ○ Intensifying contact with and sensitivity to the unborn child (awakening interest in and openness to a new and individual human being)
   ○ Group discussions and pairwork on issues relevant to parents-to-be (mother- and fatherhood, the effect of a child on everyday life; its influence on a relationship, sexuality, home- and working life)
7. Suggest various aids to breathing and relaxation which may be of value in labour. Each couple can experiment and find something to suit them.
8. Promote physical flexibility, mobility, centredness and well-being.
9. Give each individual the opportunity to express, discuss and reflect on his or her own attitudes, feelings, fears and expectations.
10. Develop trust and harmonious interplay within the couple.
11. Develop the autonomy and self-confidence of the couple – e.g., how to respect their own needs and be able to say 'no'.

12. Consider the role and needs of the man during pregnancy and birth. Reflections on fatherhood.
13. Encourage the independence and self-confidence of women and to motivate them to take an active role in creating their own experience of giving birth.
14. Use pregnancy as an opportunity for personal growth and development.
15. Build up a reasonable trust in one's birth assistants.
16. Encourage contacts within the group.

3 Rank the principles and aims listed in the box above. See which you would put first or last, give more or less weight to.
- are there any aims or principles which you don't agree with?
- are there aims which you do find important but which you don't give enough weight to in your own work?
- are there aims which you give too much importance to?
- are there aims which you have difficulty achieving?
- keep checking in the course of each antenatal class which aims get lost in this particular group and which get overemphasized.
- are there some aims which you are better suited to achieving than others? Be honest about what you feel able to give to a group.
- does this match your own priorities or beliefs about what is most important? Remember that in the end you can give more if you don't overstretch yourself or try to be an ideal 'teacher'.
- what is it that you give best?

6 Norms – values – core beliefs

In the areas of pregnancy, birth and parenthood our norms, attitudes and beliefs count for far more than all our knowledge. We all carry deep-seated and often unconscious moral attitudes and ideas that constantly affect our lives and relationships.

REFLECTIONS 1 Write down your own core beliefs about pregnancy, birth and parenthood. Try completing various sentences. For example:

- In my opinion . . .
- I think . . .
- My feeling is that . . .
- I believe . . .
- For me it is clear that . . .

Choose one sentence 'head' from the list and use it to make as long a list as possible of your core beliefs. Everything from, say, 'I believe that disposable nappies are best' to 'I believe in God'. (see Appendix)

2 Consider which of the statements you have written you feel to be simply personal beliefs and which of them you hold to have objective reality.

Check whether hitherto unconscious beliefs have come to your notice and which of these you would like to revise.

Be aware of fine distinctions:

'I think it's best for a woman to breastfeed her child.'
'I think that all women should breastfeed.'
'I think that breastfeeding is best for mother and child.'
'I think that all women are capable of breastfeeding.'

'I think that all newborn babies should sleep with their parents.'
'I think it's best for the baby to sleep with its parents.'
'I think that some babies prefer to sleep in their own beds.'
'I think that parents don't suffocate their baby accidentally if they all sleep together in the same bed.'

3 Now consider more specific situations. What are your beliefs about:
  – women who want to bear and bring up their child by themselves.
  – women who intend to hand their children over for adoption.
  – women who would send a child with Down's Syndrome to a home for the handicapped.
  – women who wanted an abortion.
  – women who need a Caesarian section.
  – women who have problems/symptoms.
  – women who show signs of premature labour.
  – babies dying during or after birth.
  – other situations that provoke definite or ambivalent feelings in you?

Be honest in writing down the beliefs you have about such situations. For example:

  ○ I believe that women show signs of premature labour when . . .
  ○ I believe that a woman who would give her child over for adoption . . .
  ○ I think that Caesarians become necessary . . .
      – when women need a way of legitimizing their wish to be anaesthetized (i.e. don't want to experience the birth).
      – when women suffer from performance anxiety (having a Caesarian then puts them in a 'special' category).
      – when a woman's sexual problems lead to rejection of her own vagina.
      – if the man finds it threatening to accept 'his' vagina being used as a birth canal.
      – when the baby wishes to avoid the pressures of birth.

Don't think of what you know or have been taught about such situations. Allow your own instinctive feelings and judgements and prejudices free expression. Don't censor your words.

There is no need to feel embarrassed or intellectually or morally censorious of the beliefs you find yourself putting down. The important thing is not to *correct* your beliefs or moral attitudes but to *discover* them. In this way they will not interfere with your professional work unconsciously.

Dealing with norm conflicts in childbirth preparation

As an antenatal teacher/childbirth assistant, how would you respond to a woman who says:

  ○ I would like to have a Caesarian
  ○ I would like to give my child up for adoption
  ○ I want to go straight back to work after the birth

(. . . or whatever it may be that runs counter to *your* norms)?

EXAMPLE

'I want to start work again after 10 weeks. Do you think it's better to get a childminder or find a day nursery?

'Oh no! You're not serious, are you?'

Or

'In fact, neither. But if anything, a childminder would be better.'

Or

'In my view, the child should be with its mother for at least the first half year.'

Which of these answers most closely approximates to what your response would be?

All three answers imply a negative judgement but the first one does at least include a definite question, and thus permits the discussion to go further. The second and third on the other hand, seal the issue and indicate that there is nothing more to be said. The answers lie like a cork on explosive questions.

With all questions that provoke value conflicts we must be careful not to answer in a way that precludes discussion of the real issues, or is blind to the real question.

EXAMPLE

'What is high blood pressure actually?'
Possibly meaning to say 'I haven't felt that well recently.'

'How often is one supposed to notice the baby moving inside?'
Possibly meaning to say 'I'm afraid that my baby might not be well.'

With some practice it is possible to get to the root of questions like this. Instead of just giving information, ask counter-questions such as: 'Why do you ask?' 'What do you mean?' 'What are you saying?' 'How do you feel?' 'Why does that worry you?' 'What are you thinking of?'

Where value conflicts are at stake, however, it is often far more difficult to be open to the question, and more self-awareness is called for. In such cases it can help to:

A six-step guide to dealing with conflicts of value

○ Breathe deeply, relax, breathe out
○ Ask yourself: How do I feel? What do I think?
○ Look at the other person. Respect her and take her in
○ Check what was meant by mirroring the question, if possible highlighting the positive aspects of her question or statement. (For example: 'You're looking for the best solution for your child given that you'll be working?')

○ Share your own feelings and thoughts honestly. (For example: 'Personally, I couldn't imagine leaving my child so soon.')
○ Ask what brought on the other person's question or statement, its background and motive. In this way check out the other person's standpoint and discover how much room there is for a dialogue that will ultimately benefit both parent and child. (For example: 'Is it definite that you will start work again after 10 weeks? How do you feel about that?')

There isn't a right way that suits everyone. All we can do is to help people to become aware of their own needs and wishes and to realize these in their respective circumstances. Putting yourself in someone else's place does not mean that you accept his or her beliefs. Nor does holding another opinion mean that you cannot put yourself in someone's place and identify with the situation.

A mother receiving a response such as the last above feels herself accepted and her question acknowledged. The fact that the teacher expresses her view clearly enables the woman to get in touch with her own beliefs and views. Now she is free to talk about why she wants to work as also to reflect upon this choice. Maybe she is afraid of not being able to handle the baby, of boredom or depression. Maybe there is social or financial pressure on her to work. None of this would have become apparent following the second and third answers. It is important for all professionals to learn to use the 1st person in their statements: to say 'I'.

Instead of saying 'You can't give your child away into the care of strangers' be honest and say 'I can't imagine giving my child away into the care of strangers'. If we hold back from expressing our personal feelings and values we hinder the individuals and groups we work with from expressing theirs.

If on the contrary we allow ourselves free and honest expression, we are by no means imposing our norms and values on the group, but simply embodying the acknowledgement that each is entitled to his or her own view.

It is not just giving our own view that is important but how we give it. It is more acceptable to others and leads to real communication if you look at the other person whilst saying directly and concisely what you feel. Far better than being indirect or longwinded, whilst at the same time showing undertones of sarcasm, aggression or manipulation.

7 Surrender and violation

The more we try to stay in control the more we fear losing control. This strain of wanting to stay in control can prevent a woman from being open, soft, and flexible during labour. On the other hand a woman can, if she wants, open herself in a thoroughly controlled way, surrendering freely with each demand her body makes.

Women who exercise perfect control during labour often reach a point at which the cervix will not dilate further. It is as if the woman cannot let go any further. At this point, medical 'help' ranges from tranquillizers to Caesarian section. Far better would be to create an atmosphere in which the woman felt free to truly let go. Dammed up fears, curses, or tears often burst forth but bring about a release and opening of the cervix.

Sometimes the body itself does the trick: the woman feels so overcome with nausea that her self-control collapses and she has to surrender – to the nausea and the release which follows. She then becomes rosy-cheeked, her eyes and lips moist, and her body soft as the cervix opens. Nausea and vomiting often herald breakdown of control and signify a *need* for release, for letting go, for surrender to the process of labour.

I am dismayed by the sort of antenatal teaching that concentrates on techniques, methods, rhythms and positions for creating a natural birth. It might be compared with an act of sexual intercourse in which, despite applying a variety of clever techniques and positions, one or both partners remain numb and uninvolved, possibly disgusted yet making nice sounding erotic noises even though it hurts.

It may look and sound like a perfect love act but, one cannot really speak of 'loving' – least of all loving oneself. It is self-violation. It is similar to someone doing Yoga, Aikido, Tai Chi, Ballet, or some form of sport without ever really getting to know the body they are 'mastering'. How much damage do we do to ourselves and our bodies in this way?

To go against the dictates of one's body (and forcefully suppress its natural urges) is to do violence to the body and to violate its ancient wisdom. Yet many women violate their bodies or allow their bodies to be violated by imposing on themselves artificial breathing rhythms or delivery positions that do not come naturally. But the role of the childbirth educator is not so much to warn or defend women against exploitation or violation, as to help women avoid self-violation. The key is in owning and trusting one's own body, this enables us not just to know what our bodies want, but also to give permission to our bodies to do what they feel to be right.

The goal is for each individual to find a personal balance between self-control and letting-be.

EXAMPLE

I felt I was really following my body's impulses well, changing my position often and respecting its every need. My breath flowed easily. The only way I felt I was still controlling myself was by suppressing my impulse to shriek and wail. I did this by switching to a controlled breathing rhythm whenever I became afraid of surrendering to this noise-making. And yet this was right for me. It was good to know that I could make as much noise as I wanted. I tend to be fairly vocal in my self-pity. That's why it also meant a lot to M. to encourage me to express this in rhythmic grunting and groaning, rather than my usual shrill complaining tone. My other habit had always been to 'lie back and wait till it's all over'. Here again, with M's help and a bit of self-control I managed to stay upright most of the time. I was pleased about this because I knew that just lying down and screaming in my usual way would have eventually brought me to the point of needing an epidural and that is exactly what I wanted to avoid.

But one will also come across women who will try to control themselves in every way and in all situations. They do not wish and are not *prepared* to give in to their bodies in any way. Yet such women can still be encouraged to treat their bodies lovingly and with care.

EXAMPLE

I was quite afraid of the pain. I'd never known anything like it and didn't think I could handle it, so I decided for an epidural. I could follow the path of the contractions on the visual display monitor. Even though I could feel nothing of it I knew my tummy was hard at work and I stroked it. It felt good to stay in contact with my body in this way. I spoke to my child, giving it encouragement after each contraction, and feeling very close to it. I don't think I could have given this loving attention had I been totally occupied with pain and breathing patterns. I enjoyed the birth of my child. Having been delivered peacefully into the world I could also receive it feeling fresh and unburdened.

The goal of childbirth preparation is not to achieve a predetermined and uniform result in all cases, but to make the woman aware of what she wants and is capable of. She also needs to be made aware of what controls she needs and the forms in which she can allow herself these.

EXERCISE

GUIDED RECOLLECTION: BREATH CONTROL

How well do you know your own body?
How good are you at surrendering to it?

Your breathing, for example:
Do you move your breath or does your breathing move your body?

Most of us experience ourselves as passive; our breathing as autonomous.

But is it so simple: breathing active, me passive?

How do you experience this being passive?
    – is it a case of deliberately not focusing on it?
    – do you stiffen yourself against your own breathing?
    – is it simply thoughtless indifference?
    – or, do you consciously or unconsciously pulsate with your
      own breath?
    – are you opening yourself to your own breathing?

What is the nature of your passivity?

Make yourself comfortable, lying or sitting.

Observe what happens automatically when your breath flows freely.

Now try another way of letting go and of being passive.

How does that feel?

This way you may discover more about your breathing and the ways it can be disturbed.

Make yourself comfortable.

Let your breathing flow just as it comes.

Now try to ignore it deliberately.

Is it possible just to forget your breathing?

How does this feel?

Now try to stiffen yourself against your own breathing.

How does that feel?

Relax again and let your breathing take its own course.

Sense the movements in your body that your breathing brings in its wake. Try to go with them.

Surrender completely to your breath.

Let it breathe you.

How do you feel?

Now breathe out and in, consciously, controlling the intensity of your breathing for a few cycles.

How do you feel?

Move your fingers and toes, stretch yourself, and let your breathing once again find its own rhythm.

EXERCISE — **GUIDED RECOLLECTION: BODY CONTROL**

Ask yourself the same question as in Exercise 1 about everyday actions of your body – eating, sleeping, walking, resting, going to the toilet.

In the course of the day do you follow or control your physical impulses?

At the moment for example, are you sitting the way your body wants to?

What determines the type and amount of activity you engage in each day. Does your body have a voice?

Who gives in to whom?

Who is ignored or repressed?

How 'democratic' are you in listening to your physical impulses?

How and who (which part of you) decides which impulses to follow?

Do you trust your impulses only if they are reasonable or do you trust that they *are* reasonable?

Consider sexual intercourse.

How do you experience it?

Of course this varies but there are parallels to be drawn with giving birth. Sex also involves breathing, positions, activity and passivity of one's body etc.

Do you tend to be active or passive?

Do you control or surrender yourself?

Do you violate or are you violated?

Passivity can be just as powerful as activity: birth is the classic example, for here we surrender to and thereby become a channel for, powerfully great activity.

It is not bad for women to take the lead or to steer their own bodies: so long as they are true to themselves.

We can use our everyday experience of being with our bodies as a natural preparation for childbirth.

– It is not the role of childbirth preparation to promote a particular ideal and establish this as the goal that all women must be trained to reach.

– The diagram should be seen as serving diagnostic rather than therapeutic or ideological goals therefore

– As a course leader it is important to know:
where you place yourself on the chart
where others would like to place themselves (their point of origin and desired destination)
what I feel about this
how to deal with groups of varying composition according to the chart

– It is not necessary to DO anything with the chart.
It is enough if it feeds our perception of the make-up of a group and our own reaction to this

– Beyond this it can also serve the purpose of making individuals more aware of the range of possible attitudes and their own approximate standpoint or position *relative* to the various classification.

– This is then usually enough to set in train a natural movement of attitude along either or both possible vectors (up/down, right/left) see figure on page 33. Or else it will help the individual to accept where she stands, even though a seed may have been planted that will ripen in years to come.

ATTITUDES PREVALENT AMONG ANTENATAL CLASS PARTICIPANTS

100% Need for control
  ○ Believe in technology. Want a technically assisted birth (induction, epidural, Caesarian etc.).
  ○ Want a rational and 'civilized' labour and accept aids to that end (pain killers, episiotomy etc.).
  ○ Want an up-to-date (fashionable?) labour guided by modern methods (Lamaze, Leboyer). New ideas and positions (e.g. standing, squatting, massage) are taken as 'musts'.
  ○ Plan their labour in the light of their circumstances. Have a definite image of how they would like it to go, but are prepared to be flexible and accept a certain element of unpredictability.
  ○ Are well-prepared all round. Have everything organized. Feel able to cope and ensure that needs are met in all situations.

50%
50% ○ Are prepared to both assert themselves in the birth situation and to go along fully with the experience.
  ○ Are well-prepared, tuned into themselves, and open to the experience of labour. Are confident that no matter what the circumstances or situation they can trust their bodies and its signals and give over to it.
  ○ Are well-prepared, know what the woman's body wants, but do not necessarily trust or follow the woman's impulses and instinct. Under optimal conditions (a good clinic or home birth) they would find this easier, but will be helpless in a technological hospital environment. On the other hand, they will not search for another hospital and neither do they actually want a home delivery.
  ○ Go to antenatal classes but do not really believe in them. Religious upbringing: women are there to bear pain. Cling to authority: doctor and midwife know best.
  ○ Are unprepared and helpless in the face of everything: technology, authority, pain and pleasure.

100% Readiness to surrender

Different mothers' attitudes during birth

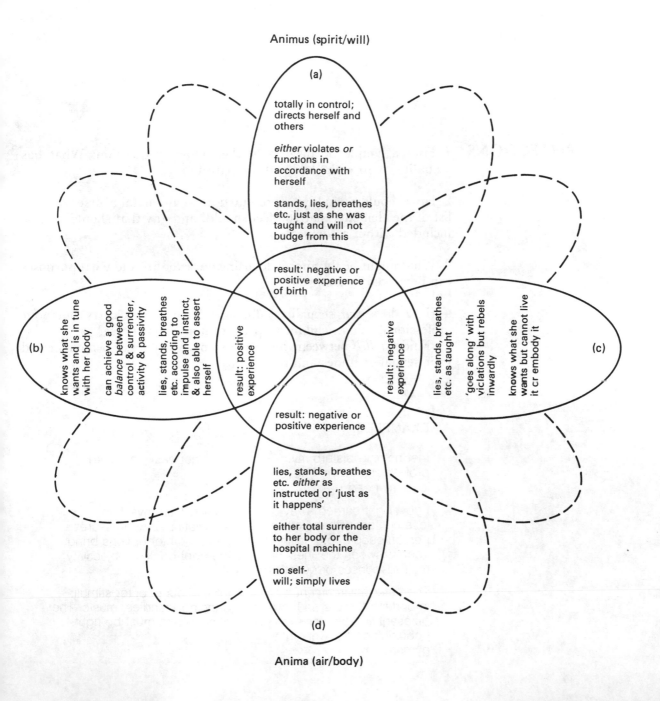

Animus (spirit/will)

(a)

totally in control; directs herself and others

either violates *or* functions in accordance with herself

stands, lies, breathes etc. just as she was taught and will not budge from this

result: negative or positive experience of birth

(b)

knows what she wants and is in tune with her body

can achieve a good *balance* between control & surrender, activity & passivity

lies, stands, breathes etc. according to impulse and instinct, & also able to assert herself

result: positive experience

result: negative experience

lies, stands, breathes etc. as taught

'goes along' with violations but rebels inwardly

knows what she wants but cannot live it or embody it

(c)

result: negative or positive experience

lies, stands, breathes etc. *either* as instructed or 'just as it happens'

either total surrender to her body or the hospital machine

no self-will; simply lives

(d)

Anima (air/body)

8 Sexuality

REFLECTIONS **1** Find a couple of answers to the following question: What has sexuality to do with childbirth preparation?

2 How should sexuality be presented in an antenatal course? Make a list of the elements that you feel should, and any that should not, be included within a course.

3 What might be the aims in focusing on sexuality and what purposes can be served in doing so?

4 How does *your* sexuality influence the way you carry out your professional role in childbirth preparation or assistance?

Find *parallels* between your professional attitudes or behaviour and your sexual attitudes and behaviour.

EXAMPLES

I let nothing disturb my professional calm. I never lose my head.

I never get carried away or lose contact with the other person/people (e.g. failing to 'read between the lines' of their responses or questions).

The outer environment is important: flowers and pleasant lighting, for example. I couldn't do my work in a gymnasium.

I am not easily aroused

I never lose myself in stimulation; any pressures, pains or interruptions bring me right back to objectivity

I need lots of outer stimuli: dancing, candles, music. The atmosphere must be right.

5 What do you wish for sexually from your partner? Make a list of quite concrete wishes, either secret ones or ones you may often have discussed. Which of them have been fulfilled? Which not?

Sexuality and birth have a lot in common: receiving; opening oneself; surrendering. There are parallels, too, in the intensity of breathing; in the moaning and groaning; in the whole experience. Indeed, the same organs are involved!

Sexuality belongs, naturally, to the subject of childbirth preparation. It should not be ignored, suppressed, or overemphasized, but in order to approach the subject meaningfully and carefully it is important to be aware of and come to terms with one's own sexuality.

Open discussion, the teacher's exemplary sighing and breathing, and encouragement of sex during pregnancy can all help to free people from inhibitions. On the other hand they can also release fear: 'I can't do it (as well as the course leader or other participants) so my labour will be difficult'.

Sex is permissible right up to the beginning of labour. But this needs to be pointed out tactfully: a woman who has little interest in sex, for example, and who has hitherto comforted herself with the notion that after the fifth month sex is taboo, is likely to feel betrayed as the rationalization for her behaviour is taken away. The result is that her trust will be weakened and further defences go up.

If the subject of sex and/or sexuality is brought up by an individual or the participants of a group you may read between the lines and find one or other of the following to be the unstated message:

○ I don't get an orgasm
○ I can't make noises
○ I get no pleasure from sex (*ergo*: I'm not normal, natural birth isn't for me)

One way of responding to this is to raise further questions for discussion:
  – is it really true that a woman who is good in bed is good in giving birth?
  – is it true that a woman who has lots of orgasms will also get pleasure from birthing?

Obviously, as course leader, you will need to be aware of your own attitude to these questions – as well as being prepared to change it. It is not always the case, but sex *can* be a good preparation for childbirth. And if you feel that a couple or the group will accept it, you can suggest, as homework, that they use sex as a natural form of childbirth preparation: by experimenting with breathing, sighing, sounding, surrendering, opening, allowing pain, positions and pelvic floor exercises etc.

A woman who had never had an orgasm and found pene-
tration very painful started using the breathing she had
learnt on an antenatal course. Her partner recognized the
rhythm, asked her if it hurt, and gave her loving attention.
From then on she breathed with the pain. Through the
intensified breathing and because she felt heard by him she
achieved orgasm for the first time.

The ability to enjoy sex can be a condition for a good birth but is
not a necessary one. Women can follow their bodies very intuitively,
opening themselves for the child and attuning to their own primal
femininity even though they may not be able to do this with their
partners. (That this is so may be a product of unconscious attitudes to
men, or may simply lie in the fact that the couple have difficulty in
communicating sexually with each other.) It is up to each couple
themselves however to determine how and how far they wish to
explore their sexuality. Overt sexual problems may come to light in
which case the couple should be firmly but tactfully encouraged to
seek appropriate professional guidance – e.g. through Marriage
Guidance.

Sexual problems associated with the first weeks, months or years
of parenthood are not uncommon and should be discussed. For
example:

*Inner and outer changes
affect the sexual
relationship*

o The father's jealousy of the attention shown to the child
o The sexual disinterest of women, whose contact needs are met
   by the child, particularly in breastfeeding
o The sexual rejection of the man, if he does not show enough
   interest in childcare or housekeeping, or if the labour was
   difficult, the child unwanted, and there is fear of a new
   pregnancy
o The inability of the man to experience the woman as a sexual
   partner after he has seen her give birth, or now that she has
   become a mother
o Infrequent intercourse due to disturbed nights, baby's crying,
   having less time together alone or opportunity to go out
o Difficulty of the woman in feeling herself to be 'sexy' and
   desirable when she has no time to concentrate on herself – to
   exercise, do her hair, have a relaxing bath, dress attractively . . .
o The effects of a painful episiotomy, sore and sensitive breasts or
   nipples, and a dry vagina (a hormonal result of breastfeeding)

There are few couples whose sexual relationship is not disturbed
to a greater or lesser extent by the birth of a new child. In antenatal
classes, especially with couples having their first child, one cannot
expect these issues to surface by themselves. The participants do not

usually anticipate such problems, and live in hope that existing problems will disappear after the birth. What is the task of the antenatal teacher? To explain? Warn? Take their hopes away? To deal with possible problems beforehand and thus prevent them? In my view our role is no more to guarantee that no future sexual problems arise than it is to solve existing ones. What we can achieve is to raise discussion, first within the group and then, ideally within the couple, and encourage each person to take her/his own needs seriously and to learn to express them. In this way, antenatal teachers can prepare couples to understand that the problems and conflicts they may experience are normal for a young family. They are not exclusively *their* problem and certainly not just *his* or *her* problem. So long as they are then able to *talk* about the difficulties that arise, frustrations will be eased and the path cleared for changing the situation and emotional responses it provokes.

SEXUALITY: A SUMMARY

– what should be discussed?
– with what objective?

1. Reassurance:
   - Dissolving false norms, preconceptions and beliefs (each couple may make love as, and as often as, they like)
   - Acknowledgement and respect for individual needs (yes to saying no! Individual needs are OK)

2. Understanding:
   - Every couple has its own frustrations
   - Sexuality is always in process and needs vary and change.
   - Different needs that men and women express

3. Preparation for birth:
   - Sex as a psychological preparation and aid: letting go, opening oneself, surrendering etc.,
   - Sex as physical preparation and aid: stimulating vaginal blood circulation (which increases suppleness for birth); stimulation of the clitoris and breasts (releases hormones which can induce and increase contractions); stimulation and ripening of the cervix due to prostaglandins
   - Preparation for changes/disturbances in the couple's relationship with the birth of the family. Discussion of possible problems. Joint acceptance of the child before it is born. Not behaving as though there were no child/no swollen abdomen.

Exercises on sexuality will be found in Part 3.

9 Fathers in antenatal classes and during childbirth

Historically in our culture, the woman's partner and father of the child has been largely excluded from the birthplace. Today, the presence of the father during labour and birth is seen as an integral part of the childbirth experience. How natural is it really?

How *necessary* is the presence of men at birth? And for whom:
– for the woman? As protector or mother-substitute?
– for the midwife, as assistant (personnel shortage).
– for himself, in order not be excluded?
– for the child, as foundation stone for their relationship?

Before we go on to set goals or exercises in antenatal classes we need to check out our own attitudes.

REFLECTION 1 To what extent do you find the presence of the man as birth attendant
– necessary?
– helpful?
– disruptive?

Write down your own chart before looking at the example on page 39.

A chart like this can be elicited from the group as a whole or the group can be divided into men and women, each group doing its own chart.

Three things to bear in mind:

1 Seeing the necessity of the man's presence at birth can remotivate the couples in preparing for birth together and attending classes together.
2 In considering the points that arise in the 'helpful' column it is important to ask whether it is only the man that can provide this help (as against midwife or girlfriend for example).
3 The points in the 'disruptive' column speak for themselves. Precisely because of this they make it unnecessary to pinpoint or isolate particular men in the class.

EXAMPLE
PRESENCE OF THE MAN AS BIRTH ATTENDANT

Necessary?	Helpful?	Disruptive?
o The shared experience of birth lays the basis for family life: – relationship with the child – understanding of the woman – not being excluded o If the woman needs emotional support o If the midwife has no time or lacks warmth o The man's presence is sometimes essential to prevent unnecessary interventions or rough treatment (the 'witness' function) o . . .	o Protection from intervention (knowing he is watching out for her, allows the woman to relax into herself) o He can speak *for* her, allowing her to concentrate on herself? o He can supply cushions and refreshments o He can massage, stroke, hug, and support her o He can provide encouragement and distraction during a long first stage o He can remind her of breathing patterns o He can suggest positional changes or supports o He can hold her upright during second stage	o Can sour the atmosphere or relationship with the midwife by being argumentative o Can be dominating/ overprotective o Can intervene and disrupt the woman's natural process o Can transmit his own fear and tension o Can massage the wrong places at the wrong times o Can urge the woman to control herself when she really needs to let go o Can encourage inappropriate breathing o Can criticize or demotivate o Can be himself more interested in the technology, monitors, etc. o May need attention himself to deal with his feelings o . . .

Do men have to be helpful?   When I introduce 'the role of the man' as a theme in my classes this is certainly not in order to 'set the men straight' on what they should or shouldn't do, but rather to encourage reflection through thoughtful questioning:

The woman is not the only one who is pregnant. Fathers too, can go through a psychic pregnancy as they accept and incorporate the changes that are on the way. Men often develop physical symptoms in early pregnancy and around the time of birth. This is their way of giving physical expression to their 'pregnancy'. Men are often expected to suppress their emotion, anxieties and pains, and their own 'labour' in order to be fully supportive of the woman.* It is useful to ask what *are* the expectations of the father during pregnancy and

*He has to take an aspirin for his headache so that he can help her to a drugfree labour.

childbirth, whether the man is obliged to fulfil them, and what happens when he doesn't. Men must be freed from this idea that they must help, and their own needs for attention and preparation need to be recognized.

Here are some examples that may aid reflection on this issue:

A   *A couple have planned a hike in the mountains. She has studied the maps, packed their rucksacks properly and so on, now they are on the mountain. A storm breaks out. There is rain and fog. Who will take charge? Who will take decisions? Who will help who over the rushing stream, the narrow footbridge? What would the answer be in your relationship?*

B   *A couple goes sailing. They have done a sailing course, though he only attended half-heartedly. They find themselves in a storm. Who takes control? What do you expect from yourself and your partner?*

A strenuous hike. Sailing in strong winds. Birth. All three are situations in which we are challenged to reveal our strengths and weaknesses, and to accept them. But if we place expectations on each other that are not fulfilled – 'Surely now he will . . .' – 'Why isn't she doing anything . . .' – a gulf opens, and with it a feeling of being deserted.

Men have individual needs too

It can also be useful to read out to the class a variety of birth reports showing different reactions from the men involved:

Gerald: 'I was really pleased that we'd invited Jane's best friend to the birth. It was as though I was lame and unable to give any practical help. Throughout the whole labour I had this incredible headache that then vanished at a stroke when the midwife placed my son in my arms. To me it was as if we were so close physically during the birth that the whole physical side of it was just too much for me.'

Andrew: '. . . I felt totally pushed to the side. The midwife, her trainee, two of my wife's girlfriends . . . they all seemed to know what to do without my help. There was this constant business, this continuous coming and going. I stood in the way, not knowing what was happening. I didn't belong there as a man. Someone brought me a sweet cup of tea. I don't take sugar in my tea! It sounds trivial but this brought tears to my eyes. I felt unacknowledged and abandoned. I really thought birth would be a joint experience between my wife and myself. She seemed to have completely forgotten about me.'

These two reports demonstrate how differently men can react in similar situations. Note also the following:

Nina: 'During the antenatal visits I had established a good relationship with my midwife. My husband had also met her and liked her. I don't know if it was jealousy or what . . . but during the labour he seemed all of a sudden to get irritated about her. He found her crude and intrusive, and began talking to me in French . . . not our usual everyday language . . . in order to screen her out, although this didn't come naturally to me. We started going from room to room, avoiding her whenever her presence became too much for Herbert. I thought he was overreacting. I was concerned not to lose her good will and didn't want to annoy her. Luckily everything went well, despite the fact that in the second stage, when she asked me to lie down so that she could monitor the baby's heartbeat, Herbert just wouldn't let me go. Somehow she respected his strong will. But I had mixed feelings about it. Our birth experience had become his. He determined the course of things, leaving me in the position of follower. I managed all right . . . but what if I hadn't?'

It takes two to tango Was he then the interfering party, the guilty one? And things could also have turned out as below:

'I noticed Herbert getting jealous of the widwife, and for a time I felt torn between them. I wanted her close, but I didn't want to hurt Herbert. Then he began to speak to me in French, the language of the country in which we had met and spent many holidays together. It was like a magic that enveloped and held us together. Suddenly the midwife seemed far away and unimportant. The birth was a dance, between Herbert and me, and I could live it fully – without being able to say who was leader and who was led. We were like a loving couple in a restaurant, with the midwife being the waiter who would occasionally bring something to our table or clear it away. This was a very important experience for our relationship, and I am grateful to Herbert for getting me to concentrate on him. As a result the birth was really a joint achievement of ours, independent of outside help. Maybe the midwife was a bit hurt. Or maybe she really understood. But then it's not her I will be living with for years to come.'

It could have also gone like this:

'After he had begun to speak French and to coax me from one room to another so that we could be alone I told him not to be so silly and that I needed the midwife now. Then he withdrew into himself and it was obvious that he was hurt. But I couldn't spare so much concern for his feelings, for I had enough to do with myself. He still accuses me today for excluding him. It was a critical point in our relationship, in which things started to go wrong.'

One could think of yet more variations to the story. But they all show how important it is to consider the relationship between man and midwife during labour. Acting out the variations using role plays would be one way to bring this out in a course.

Many men find it difficult to understand why some women in labour should feel such a need for the presence of another woman.

Why do women want another woman there?

Is it:
– a primal need?
– Because birth is women's business?
– Because only another woman who has been through a birth can understand?

What other reasons can you think of?

So what role does the husband have?

There is a difference in focus and expectations between men and women. Generally the man is more focused on the child. How will it be? Who will it be? Birth represents his first chance to see, feel, and hold his child. As for the woman, she has already been 'with child' for nine months. Her feelings are not primarily oriented to the child. She is mainly occupied with herself. Will I manage it? Men often forget . . . and how can they know . . .what an unimaginable wonder it is to open yourself to the passage of another human being into the world. Women, however, may lose sight, in the intensity of their labour, of the fact that the father, too, is involved. In this sense men can fulfil the important function of maintaining emotional contact with the child that wants to come out.

It is the woman's relationship and closeness to her own body that is reflected in her desire for the understanding presence of another woman. It is the man's relationship to the child that gives him a role which midwives, girlfriends and even the labouring woman herself cannot always match.

There are two additional points:

Why is it necessary to address all possible conflict situations?

1 In previous examples it has been assumed that the birth goes normally and without complications. But as conflicts and psychological tensions affect the birth process itself there are other variations to be considered:

EXAMPLES

– The man wants to be in charge . . . the woman fights against it . . . her cervix will not dilate any further . . .
– The man is excluded . . . the woman allies with the midwife . . . but her contractions weaken . . .

The possibilities are endless.

To make this clear in the classes can hinder the emergence of tensions, help in exploring their causes, and promote tolerance and sensitivity if tensions do express themselves during labour . . . it might need a cleansing shouting match or that the person causing the disturbance leaves the room. One task which midwife, man and women helpers all share is that of creating as relaxed an atmosphere as possible . . . one in which the labouring woman really feels she can open herself. To make sure that no sort of interference – physical, psychological, or technological – disturbs the natural birth process.

2 Pregnancy, birth, and the birth of the family are crisis times for every relationship. They are also good opportunities to take note of negative patterns that may have crept into a relationship and at least to begin to deal with these. This can be rehearsed in the final week of pregnancy and achieved during birth itself. The resulting change in patterns of behaviour can mark the beginning of a new, authentic and satisfying phase in the relationship: a new basis that will be much needed, and much tested, in the years to come. It is not a question here of giving marriage counselling or couples' therapy. The issues raised will all be closely bound up with pregnancy and birth. And yet they will also be symbolic of the relationship as a whole and of patterns of everyday behaviour. It is up to the couple themselves to 'translate' this significance for their everyday relating.

As an antenatal teacher I know that in the last analysis it is not up to me to decide whether and how much anything changes in the couple's relationship. Some couples will make a new start, some will just not listen when the issues are raised, and others, though they listen, will simply harden their position to one another.

REFLECTION   **2**   The following questions are to help clarify attitudes to the role of the father in labour, and to increase your openness to all the possible variations.
 – what does the woman want/need from the father/her partner?
 – what does the father want/need?
 – what does the father want to give and what is he able to give?
 – what are realistic expectations?
 – what are possible areas of conflict and how can these be avoided?

There are two basic attitudes a birth attendant can take and even though he is giving his best it might not meet the woman's need. She might want a more paternal when he is prepared to be 'maternal' and vice versa.

 ○ Paternal role
   – shielding, controlling, protecting woman from interference, helping with breathing and contractions.

– giving conditional support: 'I'm here but you must do your bit' or else . . . I won't like you anymore

. . . I'll be helpless and won't know what to do'

o Maternal role
– hugging, stroking, being fully there and giving his all.
– giving unconditional support:
'Whatever happens and whatever you do I'll be there for you giving support'.

EXERCISE

┌─ **WAYS IN WHICH THE PARTNER CAN HELP DURING LABOUR** ─┐

These include

o Acting as spokesperson
– freeing the mother of the need to explain or argue herself
– enabling the mother to concentrate completely on her body

o Reminding/prompting to:
– to breathe out fully (before, during, and after contractions)
– let out sounds while breathing out
– groan in deep, open tones
– check her position in terms of gravity, relaxation, rounded back etc.
– request an internal examination before any intervention
– that the next contraction is due (keeping an eye on the watch or cardiotocograph)
– (during first stage) let go
– (during transition phase) not give up, it's almost over
– (during second stage) breathe, loosen her pelvis and relax, only pushing when she feels the urge to
– remember the child about to be born!

o Offering positive feedback
– giving
– cheerleading
– encouragement
– affection
– unconditional support

o Monitoring
– individual feelings
– needs
– breathing
– degree of relaxation
– strength of contractions

o Accepting and respecting all the woman says she feels

o Helping relieve pain by:
– adjusting her position
– cooling or warming her
– providing sponges, flannels, an arm or a hand to suck
– taking the pressure off (e.g. allowing her to hang on him)
– giving massage or touch relaxation

Build up a list like this in the group or distribute photocopies. Every man and woman can tick off items: what he wants to give, what she wants to receive. Similarly, items should be crossed out: what he doesn't feel able or willing to do; what she doesn't want. Key points to discuss are those that receive both a tick and a cross. Elaborate on the importance of being able to say 'No' without guilt.*

REFLECTION   **3**   Look at all the pair exercises that are included in your course, and ask yourself:

    – what is the purpose of the exercise?

Is it to:

    – make sure that the woman receives some relief/attention that she might otherwise not get (for example because she can sit leaning against her partner)

    – teach the father a particular technique (massage, breathing awareness etc.)?

    – sensitize the partners to one another (reflection or awareness exercises)?

    – involve the father so that he doesn't feel in the way (e.g. in physical exercises for the woman such as pelvic rotations)

    – address a theme of special relevance to the fathers?

Do you find that many of your pair exercises share the same objective? If so, does this reflect your goal for the course as a whole? The same pair exercise can have several different objectives, but it is important to know how you see its purpose: an exercise with little value in teaching a technique may well be of value as a sensitization exercise; an exercise that only involves the fathers so as not to leave them out might well be used more effectively to provoke the issue of their feeling left out.

EXAMPLE

Women do the splits against the wall. The men sit with nothing to do. Some are bored, others embarrassed or irritated. They may start comparing . . . 'My wife's doing better than her', urging on . . . 'Make a bit more effort', or be concerned that the exercise may be too much of a strain.

It is worthwhile mooting these possible reactions in the group without necessarily demanding explicit feedback from the men. Often this is enough to raise discussion, and will certainly allow fathers to take stock of their own reactions and consider them in their own time.

*Remind them that this is an exercise in communication. At birth she might want something else just as he might be prepared to give something else.

REFLECTION   4   Make a list of objectives for
– the men on the course
– the couples

This need not match the model below. Before you read it, check if your own objectives match your goals for the course as a whole and the content and exercises it includes.

SOME OBJECTIVES FOR THE FATHERS ON AN ANTENATAL COURSE:

○ Sensitization to their own needs (acknowledgement and acceptance)
○ Support in being honest and authentic
○ Encouragement in deciding whether they want to be at the birth and if so what role they feel happy in taking
○ Help in dealing with the experience of being the father but also a birth attendant and expected to give help and support
○ Sensitization to the needs of the woman and to her body signals
○ Open discussion of how his partner is coping with pregnancy, birth and the newborn
○ Preparation for the extraordinary experience of birth (information, birth reports, slides, pictures)
○ Preparation for parenthood (discussion, anticipating and role-playing situations etc.)
○ Practical tips and exercises on how to help during birth
○ Cultivation of self-awareness and avoidance of behaviour that might be disturbing (pointing it out, discussing, giving feedback)

Some objectives for the couples

○ Sensitive understanding, patience and respect
○ Open communication (honesty, ability to say 'No')
○ Clear expression of expectations and needs (finding out what they want and expect from themselves and each other and the relevance this has for their relationship)
○ Clarification of the strengths/weaknesses/problems that birth and parenthood may bring out of them
○ Cultivation of awareness of individual strengths and weaknesses, and encouragement to resolve own problems

10 Dealing with pain

'Your pain is the breaking of the shell that
encloses your understanding.'

The Prophet, Kahil Gibran

Most women have an expectation of pain in labour and during their
pregnancies some will be anxious about how they will cope and what
the pain will be like. Pain is a highly subjective experience, and pain
of childbirth an emotive topic – some believing that just talking about
it can render it a self fulfilling prophecy. So that couples have realistic
expectations and are well prepared to cope with varying degrees of
discomfort and pain, open discussion should be encouraged; this will
also allay unnecessary fears and provide a basis for constructive
support.

Before attempting to teach, counsel or advise others on how to
deal with pain (whether physical, psychological or just the *fear* of
pain), it is important to be aware of your own personal attitudes and
beliefs about pain as these will inevitably colour your approach to the
topic and the non-verbal messages you express.

REFLECTIONS **1** Write down any words, images, sentences, symbols that come to
your mind when you think about pain. Don't judge, write every-
thing down, let your mind wander freely.

Now look at your associations:
Which word came first? Does this mean anything to you?
What came repeatedly in different phrases?
Are there specific situations associated with pain?
Do you want to look at them more closely?
What was missing in your own associations?
What are your blind spots?
You will find a comprehensive list of associations on page 190.

2 When someone complains to you of a headache:
Do you:
- tend to offer an aspirin?
- ignore or belittle the pain?
- compete?
- suggest possible reasons?
- suggest a lie down or a rest?

What is your most likely reaction?

3 When someone begins to cry in your presence:
Do you:
- take the person in your arms and/or stroke them?
- maintain eye-contact but refrain from touching?
- offer a handkerchief?
- offer sympathetic and encouraging words?
- ignore them and change the subject?
- tactfully leave the room to give the person a chance to recover?

What is your most likely reaction?
Are you happy with it?
Is it a reaction likely to make the person stop crying and is this what you want?
Does it correspond with the way you actually feel in such situations?

For example: You have been silently suffering under the strain of a backache and are fed up with this person going on about his or her headache. Nevertheless you offer a massage.

Or: You would really like to take him or her in your arms but don't dare and instead leave the room.

Do you react in the way that you feel you want to or do you do what you feel is expected of you even though it makes you feel uncomfortable?
How do you feel about your usual response?
There are no right or wrong reactions, all that is important is awareness of your own feelings and being free to choose to respond in a way that feels right for you and appropriate for the other person.
    Now let's look at these situations from another angle:

4 What sort of response would you yourself appreciate?
If you were crying or had a headache would you:
- expect others to be there for you and do the right thing without you having to ask for it?
- allow yourself to let go completely, become dependent, accept help from others?
- tend to push yourself on regardless of your pain/sadness/headache and deep down expect the same from others?

5 Do you look for meaning in your pain?
  - Do you need to slow down – get more exercise – take better care of yourself?
  - Do you need pain to allow yourself to rest or to get attention?
  - Do you believe there can be pleasure without pain?

6 When someone complains of a headache or backache in your antenatal class
Do you feel:
  - guilty, got at?
  - responsible?
  - challenged?
  - expected to relieve or cure that person?
  - irritated that anyone should feel anything but well in your class?

7 When someone in your group starts crying
Do you:
  - give her/him the opportunity to share the distress?
  - hold them in your gaze with caring support?
  - look distractedly out of the window, at your notes or helplessly at the other participants?
  - realize that if you take someone who is crying in your arms you may be doing this because *you* have difficulty in accepting pain or tears?
  - appreciate that comforting words or the gesture of offering a handkerchief tend to stop people crying?
  - stay relaxed yourself, letting go and breathing deeply, and helping the group itself to release unacknowledged tensions?
  - feel comfortable with the way you react in this situation?
  - feel you are doing justice to yourself and to the other person?

Some people like to be held when they are crying, they then feel secure enough to let go. For others being held is inhibiting. Some people see a handkerchief as an encouragement to cry. Others see it as a signal to stop.

It is not just a matter of which words or gestures we respond with, but of how we carry them over. Crying does not always need to be encouraged. The point is to react responsibly and authentically to all participants, including yourself.

8 Do you believe
  - that contractions must hurt?
  - that every birth is painful?
  - that there are women who experience no pain or actually enjoy contractions?

9 Do you believe that
  - women should be warned of the intensity of pain to expect
  - that avoiding the subject of pain will avoid prejudicing expectations?

Time after time we hear of women coming to postnatal class reunions and asking why nobody warned them how painful labour was. The teacher, on the other hand, insists that pain was often discussed. Did it all go in one ear and out the other? Why the discrepancy in perception? It is for this reason that I lay so much emphasis on bodywork in antenatal preparation. This counts for more than mere words in preparing women for pain. (See stress exercises p. 118.)

It should also be pointed out in classes that there are women, who, while waiting for contractions to become more painful, suddenly find themselves giving birth. This shows that the expectation of pain is not always fulfilled, just as expectation of a painless labour isn't. (See Chapter 23 on exercises to deal with pain, page 189.)

11 Fear

Introduction

Our fears influence our lives far more while they remain unconscious or unacknowledged. We do not need to change fear into trust but we can deal with it constructively once we are aware what our personal fears are.

REFLECTIONS 1 Consider your fears

- As an antenatal teacher/midwife/doctor
- When you think of birth
- When you think of giving birth yourself
- When you think of childbirth preparation classes

Do you think fear is
 – normal?
 – unnecessary?
 – necessary?
 – neurotic?
 – learned?

2 Do you address the issue of fears with your women/couples or do you wait for them to raise it?

Do you anticipate dealing with people's fears or are you afraid of it? Do you think the issue should be avoided (that discussing fears increases them)? Or do you think that it must be tackled, that everyone has fears that they should look at?

It is important to handle the issue of fear consciously and with awareness. Childbirth professionals easily avoid discussing fears whilst at the same time encouraging them by the way they talk:

'You've got to be careful of that . . .'
'It's frightening how often . . .'

'The conditions in that hospital are terrifying . . .'
'Dangerous medicines . . .'
'Damaging interventions . . .'

Insensitive talk can promote far more fear than sensitive discussion of the issue. But a conscious approach to fear demands an awareness of one's own fears and of one's fear of fear; including one's fear of other people's fears.

(See exercises on fear in Part 3, page 194.)

12   Complications during labour

There is plenty of literature available on how to avoid and cope with complications. This knowledge is important for all – parents, training groups and for childbirth professionals – but also needs to be illuminated from a psychological perspective.

REFLECTIONS   **1** What do *you* think the ultimate cause of complications is?
– mistakes and interventions in modern labour management?
– neurotic structures in the woman or in the couple?
– genetic factors?
– fate or accident?

A dialogue can be built up in a group from this question. Once again, it is important for whoever guides the discussion to know where s/he stands. Do you believe, for example, that complications can be avoided? If yes, how? And which? All of them?

2 Using a variety of examples from your own experience, build up a list of possible causes of complications. At the same time create a parallel list of the ways in which childbirth preparation could be helpful in preventing these causes. Compare your list with the chart on page 54.

EXAMPLE

Factors implicated in complications during labour	How childbirth preparation can help
Physical exhaustion	Nutritional information. Guidance in acquiring self-awareness and learning to listen to and respect messages from one's body. Permission for rest and recreation
Emotional distress ○ Troubled relationships ○ Unwanted pregnancy ○ Unresolved mother–child relationship ○ Abnormal fears or pain threshold ○ Lack of caring support ○ Anxiety	Encouraging awareness and self-acceptance. Enabling couples to ask for support from partner and/or others.
Physical causes ○ Premature breaking of the waters ○ Premature or weak contractions ○ Insufficient rotation ○ Extended second stage	As above Information, choice of hospital, exercises, positions, breathing and relaxation.
Verbal intervention ○ Negative remarks, e.g. about narrow pelvis; large head, promoting exaggerated fears ○ Inappropriate commands (e.g. to push when mother feels no urge) ○ Undermining of confidence and intuition	Information about positions and examples showing the possibility of natural birth despite narrow pelvis etc. Trust in one's own body messages.
Medical intervention ○ Artificial rupture of membranes ○ Induced and accelerated labour ○ Medication ○ Continuous fetal monitoring	Information: when intervention is required and what the alternatives are.
Genetic factors	Information and counselling i.e. choice of hospital
'Fate' or 'accident'	Eliciting self-awareness through questions: – what do I want or need? – what (changes) can I allow myself? – can I/my partner trust the birth assistants?

The principal way that we can help women to avoid complications is to use our information and exercises in order to cultivate confidence, assertiveness and positivity.

A basic positive or negative attitude influences the outcome

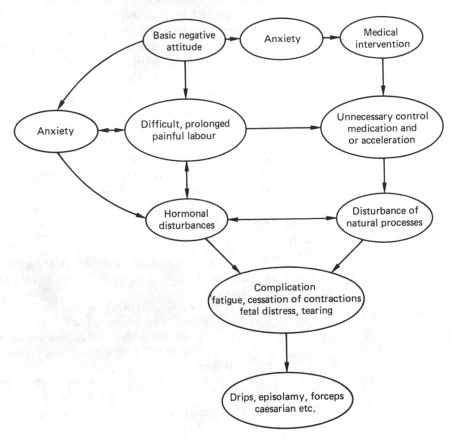

Although the exception often proves the rule within any given group of women, practically all those who choose a home birth end up with a natural labour, whereas those who choose to go into hospital experience some complication or other before, during, or after the birth. Some anticipate the complications in advance, others may choose to go into hospital because they intuitively sense them. Or is it that their basic attitude of insecurity and fear leads both to the complications and to the felt need for a hospital birth to cope with them?

Like the choice of midwife, the choice of hospital plays a big role in the labouring process. It is the task of the antenatal teacher to help women to arrive at their own choice consciously. A half-hearted decision for a home birth without a basic confidence and positive attitude brings anxiety and complications in its wake. Conversely, a good basic attitude can help bring about a good birth experience in the worst of hospitals.

Ultimately the decision rests with the individual woman/couple, whether they select a particular hospital or make the necessary arrangements for a home birth, the choice is theirs. We will not be exploited unless we allow ourselves to be; we are not powerless; pressure can be applied to the 'system' by variety of means: we can threaten to take legal action, change to competing hospitals, state our wishes in writing, restate our wishes, again, write letters to the local paper, lobby our MP; in the end it is no accident which midwife or doctor we end up with.

The role of beliefs, attitudes and choices in creating the end-result needs pointing out and reiterating, even if it is only really understood after the event. It is difficult to change someone's fundamental beliefs and attitudes in a few weeks. But we are much more responsible for the progress of labour and any complications that we may dare countenance. Our beliefs will influence our expectations, our responses and our experience.

Our beliefs can create reality

For example:

'Pain is necessary . . ..'
'The more complicated the birth, the greater the effort involved, and the greater the attention and admiration of partner and friends.'
'I don't deserve anything better.'
'Things always go wrong for me.'
'This is a woman's lot – the Bible says we must suffer in birth.'
'The system may be wrong and damaging but I am helpless to do anything about it.'
'I do not trust myself/my partner/my midwife.'

Such negative and inflexible attitudes set us up for a negative experience.

However, *expressing* negative beliefs, can be a way of acknowledging and freeing oneself of negativity, and should not be confused with attachment to it, although the two may go together.

3 Think of other similarly intransigent and damaging beliefs and the effect they might have on the progress of labour and delivery.

4 Make a list of the beliefs which you think work to define and bring out a basic positive attitude to birth.

Core beliefs work on all levels:

Buddha, who was touched by the poverty outside the palace gates, as a rich prince and who left the palace in order to seek the cause of worldly suffering, found the answer after many years of renunciation. Freedom from suffering comes only from the overcoming of longing and desire. This may have had little relevance to the beggared masses for whose sake he began his journey. It says a lot, however, about his own yearnings for the life of a prince, as he sat, cold and hungry, under his tree.

Marxism, which, like Buddhism, contains a lot of truth, could also be understood from the fact that Marx was incapable of providing for his family. His theories, which projected responsibility on the social-economic system, also freed him of the responsibility to change himself.

What is your theory that frees you of taking responsibility for the complications that happen to you – and for your life as a whole?

13 Trust

Trust is fundamental to the childbirth professional just as it is to preparation for childbirth. If we wish women to trust themselves, their bodies and the professionals and institutions handling them, then too, we must trust ourselves and demonstrate trust in others.

Trust, current practice and experience

For many years ambulant labour was viewed with mistrust; now views have changed. But the process of change required that trust be applied, and encouragement given, in the face of current practice and beliefs.

Much current practice still involves pressurizing women to push too early during second stage, rather than encouraging them to trust and wait for their own physical urge to push, and to heed and follow the natural rhythm and timing of their bodies. Many teachers pay lip service to the idea of waiting for the urge to push, knowing full well that current practice thwarts this. Like the other professionals the woman will confront during labour, these childbirth teachers have not experienced this natural instinctual urge working themselves, and therefore are mistrustful – and undermine the woman's better instincts. The fact is, however, that it is only by fully trusting that any natural process can work. Women still need to be encouraged to trust their instincts – in the face of current practice and dogma – that way positive feedback and confirming experience can be accumulated.

Trust and knowledge

The example of ambulant labour shows that the cycle of: lack of experience; mistrust; lack of encouragement for natural approaches to labour, can be broken. Knowledge, e.g. information about new research, plays an important role in breaking the cycle but may take time to become accepted. There is plenty of literature available showing, from research, the benefits of a spontaneous approach to pushing in second stage, as well as to allowing time for third stage.

This information should not be the monopoly of the teacher, but actively passed on to women to back up their active confidence in getting what they want during labour.

Trust and confidence

Trust can be thought of as passive confidence; confidence as active trust. Confidence means being able to act on the basis of trust, and to *communicate* trust through one's words and actions. It is about handling other people with trust as well as trusting oneself. It is not the same thing as presenting demands (based on mistrust) and then either fighting or resigning when these demands are not met, or when our merely passive expectations and hopes are disappointed.

EXAMPLE

A woman takes a list of questions to an antenatal check up. She can do this out of mistrust of the staff she will deal with . . . inspired perhaps by her teacher, or with a positive confidence strengthened by her teacher.

EXAMPLE

Two women: one merely hopes, the other demands that her partner will play a certain role in labour. Both women are likely to be disappointed, and both are probably unprepared for this disappointment. If, on the other hand, antenatal preparation had included opportunities to communicate with their partners about their respective needs and expectations, not only will a degree of trust have been established, but also the confidence activated to communicate needs and wishes on the basis of understanding. Instead of fearing disappointment or becoming angry, the women will be able to communicate their needs in a way that encourages their partners to fulfil them. Likewise they will be able to receive encouragement and confidence from their partners without fear that they are disappointing him.

Trust and the role of the teacher

Being a teacher or professional does not mean having to spell everything out to one's class or client. It means trusting their intelligence and respecting their boundaries. Nor is it necessary or desirable to seize upon and discuss every anxiety or problem that one senses in a group or individual. It is not what the teacher says but what she does, and the messages and confidence she communicates 'between the lines' that count. Indications can be given, and confidence imparted, but people should be trusted to deal with their own problems then, and make decisions on the basis of their own level of trust and clarity.

Almost by definition the good teacher or professional senses, sees, and is conscious of more than he or she can say. One of the principal skills of teaching is responding from this unspoken level and *taking charge* of the group process without having to either deny or spell out everything one is aware of. This is another example of trust transforming itself into confidence. The trust that unconscious and unspoken feelings can resolve themselves naturally and in their own time, that people can handle their own feelings, transforms itself into active confidence in handling the group and responding, now directly, now indirectly, to its process. But if the unspoken is a cause of self-doubt, if the teacher feels threatened by negative feelings she senses in herself and others, or if her own messages are double-edged or half-hearted, then this is what she will be communicating, whatever her words.

REFLECTIONS

1 How trusting are you?
Do you trust yourself? Your body? Your work?
Do you trust the hospitals, doctors, midwives, colleagues in your field?
Do you trust woman's innate ability to give birth?

2 Fill in all the people, events and institutions that you trust or mistrust:

Trust	++	+	+ −	−	− −	Mistrust
	myself					
					doctor B	
			midwife X			
		colleague A		hospital C		

It is useful in classes to ask participants to make up a chart like this on their own trust and mistrust. This can then be followed up by meditative questions about trust (see page 259) and one of the awareness exercises that relate to trust, e.g. 'Back to Back' or 'Tucking up and Being Tucked Up'.

3 What is your trust in the positive effects of the following:

  o Staying at home as long as possible   (1)
  o Going into hospital as early as possible   (2)
  o Having light snacks throughout first stage   (3)
  o Fasting even before labour starts   (4)
  o Being mobile, changing positions frequently   (5)
  o Resting in one specific comfortable position   (6)
  o Having friends/relatives/other children present   (7)

○ Keeping the number of those present to a minimum   (8)
○ Alternative remedies   (9)
  – raspberry leaf tea   (10)
  – arica rescue remedy   (11)
  – acupuncture   (12)
  – moxibustion   (13)
  – massage   (14)
  – icebag   (15)
  – warm water bottle   (16)
  – kissing   (17)
  – masturbation   (18)
  – breast-stimulation   (19)

○ Conventional remedies   (20)
  – glucose drip   (21)
  – Valium   (22)
  – pethidine   (23)
  – epidural   (24)
  – Entenox   (25)

○ Using a pinard's stethoscope   (26)
○ Electronic fetal monitoring   (27)
○ Rupturing the membranes   (28)
○ Lying in a bathtub   (29)
  – for most of the labour   (30)
  – for the actual delivery   (31)

○ Using
  – beanbags   (32)
  – physiomats   (33)
  – birth chairs   (34)
  – ordinary beds   (35)
  – double beds   (36)
  – delivery tables   (37)

○ Waiting in second stage until her own urge to push is felt   (38)
○ Episiotomy   (39)
○ Controlled tear   (40)
○ Injecting syntometrin   (41)
○ Avoiding injection of syntometrin   (42)
○ Controlled cord traction   (43)
○ Delivering the placenta in its own time   (44)
○ Handing the baby to the mother straight away   (45)
○ Handing a clean and warmly wrapped baby to the mother   (46)
○ Early initiation of breastfeeding   (47)

And for any given aspect mentioned above:
Have you had experience of it in your own labour or those you have attended?

Do you trust in it whether or not you have experienced it?
Do you know of any research that can back up your trust?
Do you pass on your trust in this area with or without mentioning any research results?

4 Prepare a two-dimensional chart like the one below and complete it by plotting each numbered point on the list in the position that most reflects your attitude. Then talk about it with your partner.

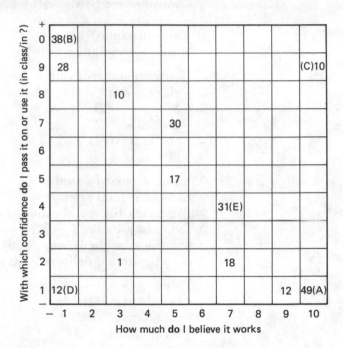

EXAMPLES

A   Waiting for the placenta to be expelled in its own time
'I believe it works but I don't dare say so in class.'

B   Allowing women to go with their own pushing urge
'I talk about it a lot, telling them about Calderyo-Barcias's research, and teaching them different positions and breathing patterns for second stage. But deep inside I am not sure if it really works because I have never experienced it.'

C   Raspberry leaf tea
'I really believe it works, having drunk it during both my labours. I make it in break time for my classes and keep mentioning its positive effects.'

D   Acupuncture
'I don't believe in its use during labour and don't mention it in class unless somebody asks for my view on it.'

E   Giving birth in a warm bath
'I really trust its effectiveness but I don't apply it very often unless the couple really want it.'

5 Can you accept that women/couples in your classes agree to certain compromises or have wishes regarding their births which, though based on their own ability to trust, may not conform to your values?

6 Can you accept that a colleague may have a style of teaching or conducting labour totally different from yours without questioning your trust either in him/her or in yourself?

Trust in one's own individuality and that of others has a good effect in classes, where women often tend to compare birth experiences and think of them in terms of 'better' or 'worse' at the expense of their own individuality and the personal differences.

In this context it is of value to consider giving antenatal classes as a pair, be it husband and wife, midwife and physiotherapist, or whatever constellation you might choose to work in.

Advantages and disadvantages of pairing up with another teacher

○ Each can specialize in a different theme, so long as they supplement each other, otherwise the course might get onesided if neither is prepared to take the responsibility for handling subjects they are both uncomfortable with.

○ Each may have different views or approaches on some questions. This is fine and can stimulate discussion, so long as neither takes a dogmatic stand.

○ Four eyes, ears etc. is better than two, so long as each takes responsibility for his/her observations and reacts to them, rather than leaving it to the other to do so.

○ If one of the teachers is a man this can help the men in the class to feel more comfortable. But teaching as a couple can also have its disadvantages (e.g. if one is more dominant or if they unconsciously create an 'ideal' example of how to behave as a couple).

○ The preparation and responsibility can be shared, though this does not mean that trust should be divided in two halves ('I wouldn't trust myself alone')

Teachers who pair up to give classes stress the advantages of having a female friend present at the birth, whereas those who lead classes by themselves stress the advantages of 'going it alone'. Women often report pleasure at having managed their labour alone without the support of a friend or even a partner. Likewise for course leaders, working alone for the first time satisfaction and self-confidence grow.

Whoever has experienced this is in a good position to work with others, contributing their own experience and self-confidence. To the same degree that our self-confidence waxes, our mistrust in others wanes. To say that I don't trust this situation or this person is to say that I don't trust my own ability to handle them.

7 Do you believe that, despite adverse circumstances (dazzling lights, noise from adjacent rooms, lacking recognition from doctors and hospitals), your antenatal courses can still be good?

Do you believe that despite adverse conditions for the participants (breech position, conflicts in the couple, technologically oriented wards, no possibilities for home births in the area etc.) their birth experiences can still be good?

Your courses live off your trust.

14 Authority and competition

The word 'authority' can evoke mixed feelings. What does it awake in you? To have authority or be an authority means more than just having qualifications or being authorized to do something. It means giving ourselves authority, and *feeling* this authority, this confidence, irrespective of our attitudes to authority, and irrespective of the professional hierarchy of qualifications and institutional rank. Do you allow yourself to be an authority in your own right (nothing to do with being authoritarian with the pregnant or labouring couple we deal with)? How can we as antenatal teachers/midwives, progressively minded doctors etc., expect to be accepted by institutions or those more conservative than ourselves if we don't believe in our own authority?

Is authority dependent on our qualifications or on whether we do our work with confidence in ourselves?

REFLECTIONS 1 Consider:

○ Situations where you
– have authority
– experience yourself as an authority
– have no authority

○ Groups of people (colleagues, parents, clients, friends, family etc.) with which you
– have authority
– lack authority

○ Who/what holds authority for you (people in uniform, doctors, judges, age, knowledge, feelings)

Think of a person who is an authority for you. What qualities does this person have that make him or her an authoritative person for you? Do you possess similar or opposite qualities?

2 Discuss with a partner or tape recorder

○ What gives you authority as a childbirth professional
○ What you need in order to trust your own authority

Speak for five minutes, beginning each sentence with one or other of the following:

'I have authority in my work because . . .'
'I am an authority in my work because . . .'

An important element in childbirth preparation should be helping women to feel their own authority and confidence. However, this is usually precisely what is destroyed during antenatal check-ups. Women are not asked how they feel and what they think. Their instinctive ability to diagnose and assess the causes of their own symptoms is given no credence, so by the time a woman starts an antenatal course her self-confidence is already undermined: she has been forced to accept the authority of doctor and midwife; and/or, she seeks a third authority in the person of the antenatal teacher. The woman is now ensnared in a net of professional opinions, and frequently advice and information is conflicting. The doctor says one thing, the antenatal teacher says the opposite, the midwife something else. The obvious result is insecurity and anxiety. An important goal of antenatal teaching must remain to increase the self-confidence of the women and couples and to restore trust in their own feelings and impulses. Some antenatal teachers do just the opposite, encouraging dependence on their own, misinterpreted, or someone else's, authority. Equally, it is sad to see how dependent women make themselves, although this may be the result of their undermined confidence. They need, or have been persuaded that they need, a good doctor, good midwife, good antenatal teacher, a girlfriend and well-trained partner at the birth, otherwise they will not manage.

But women can hardly be expected to trust themselves if even the professionals are reluctant to trust the natural birth process.

One doctor took a stand against technological birth, ultrasound scans and fetal monitoring etc. He made a name for himself in his hospital, and a lot of business for himself as a private doctor. Now when women want to book him for their births he will accept only if they have practised Yoga and on condition that they accept acupuncture treatment.

Another doctor will only attend a home birth if a paediatrician is present. On antenatal courses in which it is thought necessary to invite along all manner of auxiliary 'experts' such as obstetricians, paediatricians, midwife and breast-feeding counsellor, etc., women are bound to be left with the impression that to have a good birth they need to learn the expertise of several authorities . . . they almost need a Degree! The multi-disciplinary birth.

It may be that speakers are invited for diplomatic reasons, i.e. to improve the working relationship between the antenatal teacher and other professionals or institutions. But if this is the motive it should be made clear to the women themselves, so as not to give them a false impression of the learning required for birth.

If a woman is well-prepared for birth, confident in herself and trusting her body, it is ultimately irrelevant who delivers her, whether or not a doctor is present, etc. In the last analysis she needs no one. A good midwife will stay on the sidelines so long as the woman or couple are managing adequately by themselves. She will provide support when requested, and be on hand should complications arise. A good doctor will do the same, and not impose herself on the couple when not needed. On the other hand, if a woman is to be delivered by a good midwife or doctor does she really need childbirth preparation? Her confidence will not be undermined; she will be encouraged to breathe, sit, stand, lie, walk and push according to her own rhythm and impulse.

In this sense, the more effective antenatal teachers are in fighting for better care and conditions during labour, the more superfluous they make themselves and the more their role can turn towards preparation for parenthood. While some childbirth professionals continue to misunderstand their role as only to support the woman in her own natural process they will be interfering with birth. If they see themselves as indispensable, antenatal teachers risk hindering women from trusting and believing in their own natural abilities.

The Tower Game

An example of a group-dynamic session on authority.

Object: To build the highest, most stable tower possible

Materials: Four sheets of cardboard, one tube of glue, one pair of scissors per group.

Method: People were divided into groups of four, each group having two hours to build their tower. No observation of other groups permitted.

Results:

Group 1:   Broke up in conflict over the task. Failed to construct any tower.

Group 2:   Elected a leader. The others served as handymen, cutters, gluers etc. Succeeded in building a small but artistic tower.

Group 3:   Constructed a tower in the first half hour and spent the rest of the time taking it down and reconstructing it. Eventually ran out of glue. Returned to the large group with a plan for the highest tower, but were no longer able to build it.

Group 4:   Started off by playing cards, talking and making friends with one another. Thought that the task was less important than getting to know one another. Finally decided that building a tower might be fun and did so in the last half hour with much laughter and no hassle. Result: Not just the tallest tower but friendships that lasted right through the course.

Group 5:   Formed an organized team with discussion and division of labour. Concentrated, goal-oriented work with an impersonal and objective attitude. Their tower only fell short of winning by a few centimetres. But in their disappointment over the result the group broke up in disarray.

There are many parallels to be found here with childbirth preparation, i.e. the manner in which doctors, midwives, antenatal teachers, women and their partners come together and relate to each other. The difference is that we are dealing with the birth of a human being and not just with the construction of a cardboard tower.

15 Responsibility

REFLECTIONS **1** Are you inclined to take on a lot of responsibilities in your life? Make a list of people/areas for which you were/are responsible.

Are you inclined to avoid responsibilities in your life? Make a list of people/areas towards which you have avoided/are avoiding responsibility.

Ask yourself
- which list has the most examples?
- do the lists show how you have changed over the years?
- were there examples of situations in which you felt responsible but still avoided taking responsibility?
- were there examples of situations in which you did not feel responsible but still took on the responsibility?
- can you find examples of situations in which, in retrospect, you can now see that you took responsibility unnecessarily?
- can you find examples of situations in which, in retrospect, you can now see that you avoided taking responsibility?

2 Make lists of situations in childbirth preparation in which you think it is (a) justified, and (b) unnecessary, to feel responsible. Also ask yourself
- what am I responsible for as a childbirth professional?
- what am I not responsible for as a childbirth professional?
For example, would you feel responsible for the following?

- Changing the times of sessions/classes on request
- Being available by telephone at any time
- Phoning people when they miss classes
- Researching technical or other information in response to questions or inquiries
- Being present at the birth when requested
- Involving myself in the personal problems of clients/class members

Look at your list again in the light of 1. above
- can you detect a similar pattern?
- do you again see a tendency to take on too little or too much responsibility?
- are there situations or responsibilities which you feel ambivalent about from time to time?
- are there areas in which you take responsibility without actually feeling that you are responsible?
- are there areas in which you avoid responsibility, whilst actually feeling that you are responsible?

EXAMPLE

What do I feel responsible for as a childbirth professional?

o For my own words (and what I say with them 'between the lines')
o For my own behaviour (including my body language)
o For my own feelings (so that they are integrated enough not to interfere with or distort my encounters with individuals or groups)
o To do my best to meet the needs of pregnant women/couples on the basis of up-to-date information and all that I know

What do I not feel responsible for?

o For the feelings of the women/couples I work with
o For their decisions
o For their relationships
o As an antenatal teacher
o For interventions and complications during the birth
o As a childbirth assistant
o For births which, despite the best attention, support, interventions and intuitive guidance, go wrong

3 Think back to situations in which your responsibility was challenged to its limits. Focus on one of these situations in detail:
- who were the participants?
- what did they look like/say/not say?
- can you remember how you felt at that time?
- what do you feel now, as you look back?

Observe the situation once again in your mind:
- what was the context in which it all happened?
- what do you know about the people involved?
- what was the atmosphere - in general, and at that specific point?
- was the problem in some way representative -
    of the group
    of the individuals
    of you
- what was your life like at the time?

The exercise is intended to remind you of the many-sidedness of problem situations, and the importance of being aware of inner connections and symbolism. If you encounter a knot of problems with a group, this is one way of unravelling the knot, at least for yourself.

You are not responsible for the problems and feelings which course participants or clients have. But you are 'responsible' for how you *respond* to these feelings and problems, and for the problems and feelings that you yourself bring to your work.

Just as you cannot take the credit for a birth that goes well (can you accept that the woman did it herself and might have also managed quite well without you) so it is equally not your fault if a birth goes wrong as long as you were responsible with your feelings and information (knowledge and choice of words) and actions.

The responsibility of birth assistants
EXAMPLES

Mistakes in the handling of a labour are often responsible for the death of the baby, yet in countless examples the background reveals a couple whose relationship was only held together by the pregnancy or a pregnancy that was unwanted. Perhaps some children intend to die. Who is responsible then? We need to place our role as professionals in a broader context: one we cannot always understand or fully explain. The unborn have their own role, too, their own place, their own past and future.

1 First child. Breech position
Prolapsed cord. Midwife does nothing but waits for arrival of doctor. Lack of oxygen. Child dies. Is this the responsibility of the midwife? Background: In this family there is a history of death of the first-born going back three generations. Could the death of this baby have been prevented? Should the history of the family have been discussed and problems anticipated?

2 Second child. Woman permits a programmed labour
Contractions come slowly. Oxytocin is given in high doses. Baby is blue, does not recover and dies within a few hours. Is this the fault of the doctor?
Background: The pregnancy was unwanted. Woman in a life-crisis. In conflict with her womanhood. Unwilling to accept a child. Afraid of having a daughter, as this would intensify her conflicts.
Baby was a girl.
Could the death of this child have been prevented?
Should it have been?

We should also question the burden of responsibility that has been placed on pregnant women in recent years since the 'discovery' that the unborn child is indeed a sensitive being. The conclusion drawn is that not only should women abstain from unhealthy eating, drinking and smoking, but that they should also avoid every negative emotion of fear, anxiety or anger during pregnancy. Just as there are some doctors who would rather see unborn babies reared in incubators, so as to provide them with optimal and controlled conditions and nourishment, so there are some psychologists who would prefer to keep babies in an emotional incubator, providing only a steady supply of warmth, joy and peace. However, impurity, unpredictability and 'negative' feelings are part of normal life. The unborn bring with them their own world of feelings. They are not blank sheets, absorbing everything in total vulnerability. We should not leave mothers alone with their feelings of sadness, fear, or anger, but on the contrary, allow them these feelings and acknowledge them. The word 'responsibility' too often carries overtones of perfection: all-knowingness, pure love, selflessness etc.

'Response-ability' has to do with responding – not in the sense of giving answers to questions ('Am I doing everything right?') – but with finding an inward and personal response to the questions posed by our own, individual needs, attitudes and expectations. If we take responsibility for these, we can respond fully and ably to others, yet without having to take responsibility *for* the other person.

Doctors, midwives and antenatal teachers can carry out their duties *correctly* in every respect without being really responsible in the above-mentioned sense. The purpose of this book is to increase and deepen our ability to respond to the 'questions' of our clients/course participants, and foremost to respond inwardly to our own.

PART 2 Physiological Aspects of Antenatal Preparation

Introduction

The exercises that you will find in the following pages are meant as suggestions; there may well be other exercises that are better for you. You can choose the ones you like, reformulate, alter and combine them in any way so that they suit you and your particular class structure.

Points to bear in mind when choosing exercises for your class syllabus

o Exercises are meant to be fun: fun for you to demonstrate and for the participants to practise. There is the ill-founded belief that we only 'learn' if the experience was hard work and painful. The body and mind are much more ready to repeat an experience if it is imbued with pleasant feelings.

o Every exercise regarding breathing, relaxation and body awareness has to respect and contain the normal physical process and should never negate or suppress it.

o If you are not sure about an exercise, don't do it! Not being sure about something is usually an indication that it is not the right thing – yet – for you.

o Our bodies are what we are, and not what we have or do. There is no point in teaching or learning techniques to loosen the body (massage, yoga, belly dance etc.) unless we are open, and prepared to change inwardly.

We might *have* the knowledge and the ability to squat or keep our pelvic frame loose during labour, but as long as we are inwardly uptight, it does not matter what we *do*. It's how we *are* that influences and decides the outcome more than anything we do or have.

Whether this is the birth process, or the group process of our antenatal classes.

The scope of the exercises and my comments about them are restricted to what is relevant to antenatal teaching. There is a lot more to be found and said in the complementary areas – Posture, Movement, Relaxation, Breathing, Massage, Group dynamics etc.; see bibliography in the appendix.

16 Relaxation and body awareness

In most classes there is a large interest in and need for relaxation. It is surprising how often people will slump readily into relaxation; how those who sat tense and uptight just moments before, suddenly surrender to words and voice and to a deep relaxation – only to return into the previous tense state as soon as the exercise is over. There is no point in getting participants into relaxation if there is no learning taking place. The focus of attention needs to shift from 'relaxation' to body awareness and regulation.

The aim of 'relaxation' exercise is not so much to be perfectly relaxed as to become aware of areas of tension in the body and to practise and experience the letting go of tension. The participants learn to integrate this art of body awareness and regulation, so that they become able to recognize tensions or any sign of discomfort in their bodies without prompting, and then release the tension or respond to their needs within a few breaths. And a couple of breaths might be the timeframe between two contractions.

Because each voluntary or involuntary tensing up is an effort that uses up oxygen and energy, it is important to relax, to let go of tension during labour, so that oxygen and energy can be used more productively and not squandered. The uterus will do its task better if we relax and let it have all the available oxygen and energy.

However, a certain amount of tensing up during the contractions is normal. We might frown, tense our shoulders, hands, buttocks, thighs, curl up our toes – everybody has their own particular physical response to pain and stress. But we should let go of the tension after each contraction. If we don't, but instead let it build up, the more tense we will become and the less well our uterus will work; the contractions become more painful, we will become even more tense; and so on. It is a good rule to breathe consciously two or three times after each contraction and let any tension that has built up melt away with each outbreath.

Some labouring women feel a lot of tension inside them. It may be due to their previous experiences or to the stress of this particular labour. They seem to have great difficulty in letting go of the tension, but can be encouraged to get rid of it by walking, stamping about or squeezing a sponge etc. By doing this they are not holding on to their tension; through movement they are releasing the built-up energy that could get in the way of the flow of their contractions. It needs a sensitive partner and midwife to be aware of this, to sense when a labouring woman is getting rid of built-up energy, and when she is wasting energy. The best indicator is whether labour progresses and whether the woman is feeling well with whatever she is doing. A woman who is in tune with her body knows whether she needs movement or rest at any stage in labour.

It is important, that this body awareness and regulation is not just a technique with relevance for birth but that the participants treat their bodies, their needs, and themselves, with more interest and love in everyday life. This is also preparation for parenthood. For it is a prerequisite to caring for a newborn baby that parents are able to give loving attention to themselves and each other too.

Exercises in relaxation and body awareness

**EXERCISE
Body awareness 1**

┌─ **HERE AND NOW** ─────────────────────────

Position: Current sitting posture.
Duration: 5 min.

Close your eyes for a while and feel yourself, your body . . .

Don't change your position; just stay in the position you are now.

Now, become aware how you are feeling:
　　– how does it feel to be in this position?
　　– is this how you really want to sit?
　　– is it comfortable or uncomfortable?
　　– where do you feel tense?
　　– where do you feel relaxed?

Now, breathe deeply . . .

Allow yourself to melt into a position which feels comfortable.

Take your time.

Become aware how your body would like to sit right now.

Allow it to happen.

Observe your breathing.

Try not to change anything – that's not easy – but try . . .

Just be aware of how you are breathing:
　　– are you breathing through your mouth or through your nose?
　　– is the in-breath stronger than the out-breath, or is it the other
　　　way round?
　　– are you breathing slowly or quickly?
　　– where in your body do you feel the movement of your breath?

Place your hand where you feel your breathing movements the most.

Become aware of how deeply or shallowly you are breathing.

Breathe in deeply, then sigh as you breathe out.

Blow the air out.

Yawn and stretch yourself.

Let your breathing return to normal.

Stay in contact with your needs with any new position you might want to adopt.

Homework:　Check several times during the day while you are
　　　　　　working, sitting, standing, and before you fall asleep:
　　– how does my body feel right now?
　　– how does my breathing feel?
　　– what would I like to change?

EXERCISE
Body awareness 2

BODY PARTS

Position: Lying down, or any position with cushion/wedges under head and/or knees.

Close your eyes.

Melt into a really comfortable position.

Now, start to focus on different parts of your body. Move each part of the body mentioned to become aware of that area.

Sequence of awareness

Left leg: toes, sole, ankle, calf, knee, inside and outside of thigh.

Right leg: as above.

Buttocks, pelvic floor (tensed and relaxed).

Tummy (widened with a deep breath and relaxed).

Back (feel each vertebra along the spine pressed against floor.)

Chest (widened with deep breath, and relaxed).

Left arm: finger, hand, wrist, arm, elbow, shoulder.

Right arm: as above.

Neck (head rolled slightly).

Scalp: (tensed up and released).

Hair

Forehead (tensed up and released).

Eyes (eyelid on the eye, eyes rolled to and fro).

Nose (sides of the nose moving with breath).

Cheeks and jaws (loosened through movement; contact to the teeth, air blown through the hollow of the mouth).

Mouth and tongue (saliva; softness and roominess inside the mouth).

Breathing (focusing on out-breath; allowing body to become softer with each out-breath).

Gradually, slowly move again.

Stretch, yawn, sigh, curl over on one side, roll up to sitting position.

**EXERCISE
Body awareness 3**

┌─ **FLOOR/CLOTHING/AIR/WELLBEING** ───────────────

Position: On floor with wedges, cushions and blankets.
As comfortable as possible.

Duration: . . .?
Take your time; experiment with different positions.

Let yourself feel heavy, and feel the hard floor through the
blankets and cushions.

Let yourself feel supported by the floor underneath.

Feel yourself rooted.

Let yourself know whether you like that or not.

Remain in that position if you like it; if not experiment with
another.

Find a position where you feel minimum pressure from the floor.

Feel light and soft.

Take your time . . . experiment . . . come to rest in the position
that you feel most comfortable in.

Now, focus on the clothing that surrounds you.

Does anything feel tight, too warm, unpleasant?

Try to make yourself more comfortable.

Now feel what else you can become aware of:
  – with which parts of your body can you feel the fabric of your
    clothes?
  – with which parts of your body can you not feel much,
    although you know that something is touching you.

Be aware of how the different materials feel.

Which materials feel pleasant to you? Are there materials that feel
unpleasant?

And you can always change your position if you like.

Now, focus on the air that surrounds you.

With which parts of the body can you feel contact with the air?

How does it feel?

If necessary make yourself more comfortable.

Become aware of how the air around you enters your body and
then leaves you again.

Follow the path of the air into your body and outward again.

Experience the closeness with the air around you.

Now, focus inside yourself.

What do you easily become aware of?

Note what feels tense and unpleasant inside, and what feels well and pleasant.

Stay in contact with your whole body for a while, inside and outside.

Let your body know that you can feel all its signals; even if you might not be able to respond to all its needs just now . . .

Enjoy all that feels pleasant and good in and around your body (the floor, clothing, and the air that surrounds and supports you).

When you feel ready, stretch and yawn, and sigh; move about a bit and gradually come back into the group.

EXERCISE
Body awareness 4

INNER SPACE

Position: Lying down.

Duration: 15 min.

This exercise lends itself to repetition in class. Give less and less verbal prompting and time on each occasion, so that by the sixth session participants are able to reach the same level of openness and softness within two minutes.

Aim of this exercise

- ○ Relaxation of the whole body
- ○ To allow breathing to flow more freely and deeply
- ○ Relaxation of mouth and throat
- ○ To experience the connection between openness of throat and pelvic floor
- ○ Awareness of the spaciousness and boundaries of the body
- ○ Increasing awareness of the ability of the body to be a passage for the baby

Lie down and shift and change position until you feel really comfortable.

Find a position in which you don't need to hold any part of your body.

Take your time . . .

You are going to embark on an imaginary journey through the inner spaces of your body.

Breathe deeply and slowly, and feel the width of your chest from within.

Breathe deeply and slowly.

Imagine your breath could enter not only your lungs, but stream into the whole chest.

Try to feel the shape and width of your chest from within.

Now move your attention further up . . . along your throat and neck; imagine your neck to be an open channel through which your breath flows freely.

Move further up still into the inner space of your head; how large or small does this space feel to you? How wide or tight do you experience the inner space of your head to be?

Try to feel the space inside your nose; how narrow or wide are the passages?

Allow your breath to flow freely through your nose.

Become aware of the inner space of your mouth . . . fill your cheeks with air . . . feel for the space between your teeth and cheeks, and between your teeth and lips.

Experience your mouth as soft and wide, and then let your awareness move along your throat, downwards again, into your chest.

Allow your throat to be wide open.

Breathe deeply and gently.

Allow your breath to flow freely . . . through nose, mouth and throat into your chest.

Imagine your air passages to be like a slow wide stream.

Now move your awareness from your chest into your right arm.

Imagine your arm as hollow, and experience the inner space of your arm.

Allow your breath to flow into your arm.

Experience the inner space of your elbow, and move your awareness further down.

Feel the inner space of your lower arm, your wrist, your hand . . . and become aware of the roominess inside of each finger.

Imagine your breath to flow from your chest into your right arm, into the fingertips of your right hand.

Then breathe consciously again.

Feel the spaciousness of your chest, and move your attention from there into the space of your left arm.

Allow the breath to flow into your left arm.

Experience the shape of your left arm from within.

Experience the inner space of your elbow, of your lower arm, of your wrist.

Be aware of the inner space of your hand, of every individual finger.

Imagine your breath flowing all the way into the fingertips of your left hand.

Breathe deeply and gently.

Be aware once more of your chest, your throat, your head, your arms and hands.

Now move your awareness from your chest into your abdomen.

Widen your tummy with your breath.

Experience the width and spaciousness of your tummy.

Feel the boundaries of your tummy.

Imagine the inner space of your tummy as hollow and soft and wide.

Breathe deeply into this spacious cavity.

Experience the inner space of your pelvis.

Allow yourself to feel the opening in your pelvic floor.

All wide and soft and open . . .

Breathe all the way down into this opening and out through it.

Breathe deeply and gently.

And experience yourself as soft and spacious . . . in your chest, in your throat, in your head, in your arms, in your hands, in your tummy, in your pelvis.

All is soft and wide, your breath flowing everywhere.

Now, move your awareness from your pelvis to the inner spaces of your right leg.

Imagine the inner space of your thigh, and your knee.

Imagine your breath flowing all the way down into your right leg, into your calf, your ankle.

Experience the width or narrowness of your foot.

Feel for the spaciousness of every toe from within.

Breathe gently and deeply, and imagine the flow of air all the way down to the toes of your right leg.

Now, move your awareness to your left leg.

Imagine the inner spaciousness of your thigh.

Imagine your breath to flow into your left leg.

Experience the inner space of your knee, your calf, your ankle.

Become aware of the space within your foot, and within every single toe.

Breathe gently and deeply and experience your body as whole, spacious, wide and soft.

Imagine your breath to flow through your whole body.

Experience the spaciousness of your mouth, of your throat, of your chest . . . all the way down into your tummy, and into the openness of your pelvic floor.

Breathe gently and calmly.

Allow your breath to flow freely.

Experience the spaciousness and boundaries of your body.

Then, slowly begin to move your fingers and toes, gradually move your limbs, stretch, yawn and sigh.

Take your time and gradually come back into the group.

EXERCISE
Body awareness 5

STANDING

Duration: 5–7 min.

First, experiment with the way you can stand most comfortably.

How far apart do your feet want to be?

Try out various widths; shoulder breadth?; hand breadth?

There is a theory that your pelvic joints are most relaxed if your feet stand as wide apart as the distance between your ischial tuberosities.

Feel for your ischial tuberosities, if you can't feel them, sit down on a hard surface for a moment and wriggle your bottom. You will become aware of them and be able to feel the distance between them. It is good to know how much space there is between your ischial tuberosities as your baby will come through this space.

Try a standing position in which you create that distance between your feet. How does it feel to you?

If you like, alter the distance between your feet until you feel you have a good stance.

Now, does it feel better if your feet are parallel to one another or do you have a better stance when your toes point inward or outward?

Change the position of your feet again.

Listen to the signals your body is sending you.

Be aware of what is comfortable and what feels unpleasant and follow your own body's needs.

Now focus your attention on your legs.

Are they straight or slightly bent?

Are your knee joints locked and tense?

Try bending your knees and bounce slightly up and down.

Within a few centimetres and then millimetres, try to find just the right position for your legs – where you don't have to tense up to keep them straight and where you don't have to tense any muscles to keep them bent.

Take your time over them. Don't worry if you don't find the perfect position for your legs straight away, what is important in this exercise is to become aware of any tension and strain our bodies create.

Remember that you can always alter the position of your feet and legs as you become aware of new signals your body is sending you.

Now, focus your attention on your pelvis.

Move your pelvis forward and backward, rock it gently sideways, loosen it anyway you like – keep your feet firmly on the ground and your knees unlocked.

Let the rocking movements of your pelvis become smaller and smaller until, within the last millimetres of rocking it forward and backwards, you find the position, where your pelvis can rest on your thigh bones without any strain or tension.

You can always change the position of your feet, legs and pelvis again, to suit your needs.

Now, gently sway with the trunk of your body, feeling for the point of gravity where your spine, and the weight of your abdomen, can rest on your pelvic frame without straining your tummy or your back muscles.

Now, focus on your shoulders, move them back and forward, pull them gently up, rotate them in a forward direction, and then backwards.

Gradually find a position in which you don't have to tense up to hold your shoulders.

Find a position in which your shoulders can rest on your trunk.

Now, let your head gradually lean backwards.

Let it hang down, backwards, as far as possible.

Feel the strain and tension in your neck and throat. Observe what happens with your breathing as you allow your head to hang back.

Open your jaws and mouth.

Now, very, very gradually bring your head up again.

Very slowly, millimetre by millimetre, observe the change of tension in your neck and throat, observe your breathing, as you bring your head up again.

Now let your head slowly lower itself forward, more and more; let the whole weight of your head lean forward onto your chest.

Observe what happens to your breathing.

Be aware of the tension in your neck and throat, and just allow it to be there for a while.

Open your jaws and mouth.

Very, very gradually let your head come up again.

Observe the change of tension and your breathing, until you reach the point on the top where your head can rest on your spine, where you don't have to tense your neck to hold it.

If you want, move your head very slightly forward and backward again, until you find the position, that feels just right for you.

Now, be aware of how you are standing with your whole body.

Your feet, your legs, your pelvis, your trunk, your shoulders, your head.

Let yourself know of any tension that you use to hold yourself in a certain position and release it if you can, changing your position once more, however slightly.

EXERCISE
Centring

GLASS SPHERE

Position: Standing, knees unlocked and position of feet as comfortable.

Duration: 5–7 min.

Feel the heaviness of your body in the soles of your feet.

With each out-breath allow yourself to feel more rooted.

Imagine yourself to be a reed being moved by a gentle breeze and the water surrounding you.

Very slowly swing forward and backwards, or sideways, any way your body wants to move.

Your feet remain firm on the ground.

Your body swings and circles gently in all directions.

Don't let the movement go too far.

Let your toes be an indicator.

If your toes curl up you are going beyond your line of gravity.

Explore how far you can extend your centre.

Allow your arms to move too.

Swinging, floating gently sideways, upwards, and downwards, forwards, backwards.

Bend your knees, if you want to extend your movements even further.

Keep the soles of your feet staying rooted on the ground.

Now imagine you are surrounded by a glass sphere.

You are following the curves of that imaginary glass sphere from within.

Follow the invisible curves, upwards and downwards, sideways, in front, behind, and underneath you.

Explore your own sphere in all directions.

It does not matter how big or small your sphere is.

Only remain with your centre (let your toes be the indicator) while exploring your invisible sphere.

Allow your breath to flow with your movement.

Breathe out, as you sweep gently downwards with your hands.

Breathe in, as you let your hands glide upwards along the invisible curves.

Extend the movements as far as feels comfortable.

Remain in touch with your centre.

Then, in your own time, let the movement cease and come to a rest.

EXERCISE Centring

SORT OF TAI-CHI

Position: standing.

Duration: 10 min.

Music could be played and the participants allowed to move easily and lightly in a centred way. Movement through the room is possible as well when the lifted leg is put down in a different place.

Find a resting, relaxing position.

Feel the heaviness of your body.

Breathe deeply and calmly.

Focus on your breathing, feel the upwards and downwards movement of your breath inside you.

Allow yourself to become heavier with every outbreath.

Feel yourself become lighter with every inbreath – as if you were drawn upward by invisible threads.

Just feel the rhythm of lightness and heaviness.

Now imagine that there are balloons in your armpits: with every inbreath they become big and round; with every outbreath they become small and flat.

Allow your arms to lift away from your body with every inbreath.

And to return to your body with the outbreath.

Now, very slowly, allow your heels to lift from the ground with each inbreath, but only a tiny bit.

With the outbreath stand firm and heavy on the floor again.

Don't exaggerate: it is not important to stand on the tip of your toes while breathing in; only feel the lightness inside you.

Let your heels lift only as far as you still feel naturally balanced.

It is important, to be centred, even more so in feeling lighter.

And now shift your weight to one foot, and with the next inbreath lift the other foot off the ground just a few millimetres, only as much as your foot does by itself.

With the outbreath let your foot return to the ground.

Repeat this a few times.

Don't force anything.

Don't lose your balance.

Now shift your weight and allow your other foot to leave the ground and to return to it in the rhythm of your breath.

Now, let your legs rest.

Keep your weight on one leg while the other is resting with the knee slightly bent.

Move your hand forward, so that it is above the flexed knee in a comfortable position.

Imagine a string which connects your hand with your knee, as if you would lead a puppet.

With the next inbreath lift your hand very slowly and lift the knee and your leg with it.

Lower them very slowly.

Stay centred.

Your inner balance is more important than the height your foot could reach.

Now, try to shift your hand sideways, very slowly and take your leg with it.

Lead your leg up (with the inbreath) and down (with the outbreath), and sideways, outward and inward.

Make a circle with your leg.

On an outbreath return it to the ground again.

Now shift your weight to the other leg and feel your breath.

With the next inbreath move your other hand forward to a position above the flexed knee and . . . etc.

EXERCISE
Awareness 1

WALKING

It might be best to divide exercise into 5 sections, spread over several sessions
Duration: 2–5 min. each, or 10 min. if done as one exercise.

○ Walk around the room freely or in a large circle.

Walk on the outer edge of your feet.

Walk on the inner edge of your feet.

Put the toes down first, and let the feet roll the full length of the soles.

Put the heel down first and let the feet roll the full length of the soles.

Let the left foot walk on the toes, and the right foot on the heel.

Let the right foot walk on the toes, and the left foot on the heel.

○ Experiment with different ways of walking.

Exaggerate, soft, springy, scattered, stomping, cautious.

○ Let the shoulders and/or arms circle while you are walking.

Move the centre of your body.

Let the pelvis make circles.

Walk while belly-dancing.

○ With every step contract and relax your buttocks.

Tilt the pelvis forwards and backwards while you are walking.

Find a gait which tilts the pelvis slightly forward.

○ Find a gait where legs, pelvis, spine, shoulders and neck feel comfortable.

**EXERCISE
Awareness 2**

MOVING LIKE A NEWBORN CHILD

Position: Lying down

Duration: 5–10 min.

Curl up in a fetal position.

Stretch one leg, and then the other.

Make fists, then relax your hands.

Stretch and bend your arms, alternately.

Slowly turn on your back.

Now, draw your legs towards your chest like a newborn child.

Stretch them into the air.

Kick.

Fidget with your arms, then stretch them slowly, consciously upward.

Look at your hands, and your feet.

Rotate wrists and ankles.

Move your limbs in all possible ways.

Experiment with how you can move your limbs about.

Create a dance.

Let your arms and legs dance – in very tiny movements; in very spacious movements.

Be aware of your body.

Feel yourself from within.

Roll back onto your side.

Allow yourself a comfortable resting position.

Feel the movements reverberate in your body.

17 Breathing

Most people associate antenatal teaching with learning new breathing patterns. Is this fair comment? What role does breathing play in *your* classes? In *your* life? In *your* body?

Approaches to breathing

Most antenatal classes emphasize one of the following approaches:

1. Physical exercise, perhaps combined with information about the birth process and help available. The basic attitude is that special breathing is unnecessary: to combat pain or tension medication and obstetric care is adequate and best;
2. The prevention of pain and stress at birth through information, discussion, and assertiveness and relaxation training (choice of birth place, avoidability of unnecessary intervention). Here, the basic attitude is that special breathing is unnecessary; stress, pain and fear are all avoidable;
3. Information and discussion, and the importance of learning certain breathing techniques. The basic attitude is that special breathing is necessary, only then can we control stress and pain;
4. A combination of information, discussion, physical exercises and certain breathing rhythms. The basic attitude here is that stress, pain and fear may not be avoidable in present circumstances so special breathing is still needed.

Which approach do you follow?
Which basic attitude do you hold?
Which basic attitude are you confronted with in your environment of local hospitals, midwives, class participants?

If you consider appraisal of breathing important, which form do you give it?
- patterns?
- technique?
- therapy?
- rhythm?
- flow?

Every word holds other associations.
Which is the word connection that you use? What does this word mean to you?
Do you use the word that best conveys what you are actually teaching?

Some teachers still use the term 'breathing technique' although their style of teaching has nothing to do with imparting technique. Others speak of 'flow' or 'rhythms' yet between the lines they are dogmatic, so 'technique' would be far more appropriate.

What do you want to achieve by focusing on breathing in your antenatal classes?
Complete the following sentence:

The aim of ....* in antenatal
teaching is ....**

* insert your own word for 'breathing' (see above)
** complete the sentence with your personal aim.

It is most important that you are clear about what you want to achieve. From your aim you can derive the structure and the type of exercises you want to use. Check through your course contents. Does it really correspond to your aims? Often one reads in course syllabi of 'the body's own ability to breathe just right' yet the breathing patterns offered in classes don't allow any freedom for individual breathing rhythms.

Some breathing techniques and their uses during labour

1. Full concentration on breathing.
   Aim: No thoughts left for pain or fear.
   In practice this can mean focusing intently on evermore difficult breathing patterns, i.e. counting each in- and outbreath; remembering each level and area of the body one is supposed to reach with the breath etc; or, it could mean focusing intently on our own individual breathing; to remain meditatively concentrated throughout; to remain aware of the movement of our breath; to flow with it; to ride on it.
2. Delivering the optimal amount of oxygen to the body.
   Aim: The body is able to function unimpeded and with less pain and stress.

In practice this can mean that the optimal amount of oxygen can be provided by following certain rules of 'ideal' breathing; or, it could mean that the optimal amount of oxygen can be provided through trusting our own body signals and needs and allowing the body to breathe, to follow it and flow with it.

3. Breathing with meditative rhythms.

Aim: A trance-like state where the reality of stress and pain does not reach us any more.

In practice this can mean to aim for an out-of-body or rebirthing experience that takes us away from the actual here-and-now birth (quite often induced due to hyperventilation in transition stage); or it could mean: to aim for a trance where we are at one with our body, where we *are* body, where we *are* breath, where we *are* uterus and no longer head or mind.

The different usages of breathing offer us control or surrender depending on how we use them.

Many women expect and want to learn strict rules and breathing techniques. As they will not change their beliefs overnight, they may be offered rules and patterns (see following pages) together with body awareness exercises and encouragement to trust in their own bodies.

Practising and exploring a whole range of different patterns (see pages 95–118), will widen the participants' spectrum of possibilities and increases their awareness of *what feels right for them* and what doesn't. Some will find their own rhythm(s) or will adopt one of the patterns shown in class that they feel comfortable with and will use in labour to stay in control. Others remain totally open and trust their bodies to breathe optimally whatever the situation.

Unfortunately though, the choice for surrender or control is not just dependent on the personality but on outer circumstances as well:

A labouring woman knowing herself to be in an environment that is imposing pressures, interference and stress (be it through attitudes of those present or medication and machinery used), feels it might well be easier for her to stick to breathing patterns or techniques to stay on top of things, than to try to surrender to her body and lose her hold on her unsympathetic environment. On the other hand, a labouring woman knowing herself in a pleasant stress-free environment (hospital or home) will find it easier to surrender to her body.

In a stress-free situation the body can take care of itself and needs no patterns or techniques. But taking into account that such a stress-free environment is not always given and that some people are not able to let their bodies breathe even if they wanted to, learning breathing patterns may still be valuable.

Objectives and how to achieve them

The aims of learning breathing awareness/patterns are to acquire a breathing which:

○ Provides both the muscles of the uterus and the baby with the optimal amount of oxygen
○ Flows naturally and effortlessly, no need to exert ourselves, neither mentally (to remember a pattern), nor physically (to force a pattern that doesn't happen by itself)
○ Remains with us (or we with it) whatever the pain, stress or interference encountered

Five steps towards a breathing that flows freely and efficiently

This breathing is achieved by:

1. *Getting to know one's own breathing rhythm*; it is the foundation on which to build more free-flowing breathing
2. *Observing critical aspects* in one's own rhythm and correcting them as necessary

Some examples of maladaptive breathing and corrective measures that can be taken.

After the inbreath not to hold in the air but let it stream out again without interruption

We all tend to hold our breath in fear and painful situations. Some people have experienced so much fear or pain in their lives that they have 'learned' to breathe that way; inbreath – stop – outbreath; inbreath – stop – outbreath. In labour, this pattern would be especially intensified. During contractions the tendency to hold the breath would cause an interrupted flow of oxygen. Which means that both the uterine muscles and the baby don't get as much oxygen as they need. The same applies for the stopping after the outbreath although a little rest is more natural there. However, if it is held too long the body reacts with having to draw in air actively which is unnecessary effort.

During the outbreath not to push out more air than necessary

Some people tend to breathe out forcefully, exerting their abdominal muscles additionally to the diaphragm to push out more air unnecessarily. If the basic mixture of carbon dioxide and oxygen that should remain in the lungs, gets pushed out with each outbreath, the body will take in too much oxygen with each inbreath, causing too low a level of carbon dioxide in the blood plasma and hence hyperventilation.

Under normal conditions this might not happen, but as ingrained tendencies are usually increased under stress it could be a disturbance in labour. The other disadvantage of this type of rhythm is the unnecessary effort the abdominal muscles make with each breath. Each unnecessary strain during labour, whether tensing of muscles due to stress, or this tensing up of the abdominal muscles to 'assist' each outbreath, is a waste of energy. All the energy should be available for the work of the uterine muscles.

Do not gasp for air with the inbreath but let the air stream in effortlessly

In shock or panic situations we all tend to gasp for air. For some people breathing in such a rhythm is natural. In labour, this type of breathing pattern is likely to be increased and could lead to intensified feelings of panic. Furthermore, taking in more oxygen than the body needs could in turn lead to hyperventilation and unnecessary effort with each inbreath.

It may be worthwhile experimenting with these 'wrong' and 'right' breathing rhythms to experience the contrast:

○ Inducing fear through holding our breath after each inbreath
○ Inducing hyperventilation through pushing out too much air with each outbreath
○ Inducing panic through gasping for air with each inbreath
3. *Experimenting and practising* to let the breathing flow effortlessly in its own individual rhythm
4. *Using each outbreath consciously to aid relaxation:* let go of tension with each outbreath; let off steam, sighing, groaning actively or allowing any tension to melt away with each outbreath.
5. *Making room inside oneself with each outbreath* for new energy, for fresh oxygen (see rules below).

However much we would like to take *in* oxygen, first of all we have to create room for it inside us. The image of the shopping basket is apt:

If we go shopping with a full basket [lungs and body are full] we can't buy much [no room for fresh oxygen] so we make sure it's empty before we set out. Yet we shouldn't empty it completely: we have to leave the purse in [the basic mixture of exchange gases in our lungs].

The basic rules

○ Emphasize the outbreath without forcing more air out than necessary
○ Allow the inbreath to flow inward, without actively drawing it in
○ Allow a smooth transition from inbreath to outbreath without holding the breath

Everybody can apply these rules to their own individual breathing, however deep or shallow; fast or slow. This way of breathing effortlessly will help alleviate pain by:

○ Providing the uterine muscles with a good supply of oxygen so that they tire less, which means less pain
○ Each outbreath eases unnecessary tension in other parts of the body, shoulders, buttocks, hands, etc. They will tire less, which means less pain
○ Allowing all the energy to stay in the uterine muscles etc., as no effort is wasted on breathing

The exercises which follow show how to develop this type of breathing in class. These exercises can be varied, adapted, shortened or extended, to suit requirement and interest.

Exercises in breathing

Any exercise you do can be used on different levels for a multitude of observations and results. In groups with little awareness it is best to start with very simple exercises and build on them. In other groups you could start straight away with the awareness exercises on page 97.

**EXERCISE
Breathing observation
1**

SELF-OBSERVATION

Provide paper and pens.

Position: sit comfortably, in any position.

Observe your own breathing.

Count the length of each breath. Is the inbreath or the outbreath longer? Is there a rest after each inbreath and/or after each outbreath?

Observe the depth of your breath.

Where in your body do you feel the movement?

Put your hands there, where you feel your breathing most.

Observe how you breathe.

Do you draw in air actively?

Do you push out air with your abdominal muscles?

Place your hand on your tummy: is there any straining?

Is your breath flowing freely without effort?

Draw the pattern of your own breathing, thickening the lines where you 'help' actively.

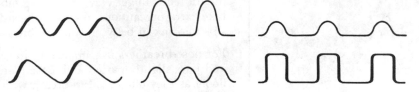

Share and discuss the observations with the group.

Sit back once more and try to let your breath flow freely – neither drawing your breath in nor pushing your breath out.

Just let it happen.

Now become aware of any changes in your breathing.

How long is the outbreath and the inbreath now?

Do you take a rest after the inbreath or outbreath?

Where in your body do you feel the movement most?

Is your breathing deeper or shallower than before?

Draw the new pattern of your breathing over the old one in a different colour.

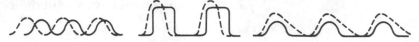

Share and discuss the observations in the group.

EXERCISE
Breathing observation
2

PAIR EXERCISE

Ask pairs to observe each other's breathing for a few minutes: A relaxes, B observes; B relaxes, A observes:
- how many breaths does each make per minute?
- is the in- or the outbreath more intense?
- does the breath flow mainly through nose or mouth?
- where can the breathing be seen in the body?

Share the observations with the whole group.

It does not matter whether one breathes through the nose or mouth. For mouth-breathers it is important to know that the mouth tends to get very dry during labour, so they will have to take extra precautions to suck a moist flannel or sponge or have sips to drink in between contractions.

For nose-breathers it is important to remember to keep their lips and jaws slightly parted and loose (connection: mouth–pelvic floor) as they often tend to breath with tight lips. Some people like to breathe in through their nose and out through the mouth. Anything is right as long as it is effortless.

EXERCISE
Breathing observation
3

┌─ **VARIATION** ─────────────────────

Ask participants to observe and count how often they breathe in one minute.

Share and discuss the observations with the whole group. The aim is to show and accept the multitude of breathing needs and rhythms.

Observing somebody else (pair exercise) can be more illuminating than self-observation, and the inhibiting feeling of being watched is common experience in antenatal and obstetric care.

Introduce the questions:
  – are you still able to relax, to stay with yourself?
  – are you able to ask for space?
  – do you feel grateful if somebody observes you closely?
  – do you feel he/she has been competent?
  – do you think your own observation would have been more accurate?
  – did being observed alter your breathing?
  – what does this imply about your antenatal obstetric care?

EXERCISE
Breathing awareness
1

┌─ **NOTICING CHANGES** ─────────────────────

Aims:

  ○ To experience the difference between free-flowing breathing and actively supported breathing
  ○ To experiment with faster and slower breathing to help participants find their own rhythm
  ○ To experience hyperventilation (not only hear about it) and what causes it and how to correct it.

Make yourself comfortable sitting or lying down.

Take your time.

Now, become aware of your breathing.

Follow the flow of your breathing, inbreath and outbreath.

How easily and freely does your breath flow?
  – do you tend to 'help' your inbreath or your outbreath?
  – do you actively suck in air with your inbreath?
  – do you actively push out air with your outbreath?

Give all your attention to your breathing.

If other thoughts pop up just observe them and let go of them with the next outbreath.

Only your breathing is important just now.

Open yourself to the inbreath, and let go, melt, with the outbreath.

Become aware of in which parts of your body you feel your breathing most.

Where do you feel most movement inside of you with every breath?

Place your hand on that area of your body where you feel most of the movement.

Stay with those waves of breath inside you for a while.

Now be prepared to experiment a bit with your breathing.

Try breathing faster and shallower than you normally breathe, just for a while.

How do you experience this sort of breathing?

What is changing in your body if you breathe faster and shallower?

Where in your body do you feel those waves now?

Try breathing a little bit faster and shallower still, very light, just like a flutter.

How do you feel breathing like this?

What happens in your body?

Now breathe out deeply a couple of times.

Let go of any tension that has built up.

Allow yourself to return to your normal way of breathing.

If you got a bit dizzy doing that fast breathing, place your hands like a cup over your mouth and nose and breathe in your own outbreath again. (This helps reduce any excess oxygen that you might have taken.)

Now, allow your breath to become deliberately slower and deeper than normal . . . and then, a little bit deeper and slower still.

Feel for the waves of your breathing in your body, and with every breath try to reach further and deeper into your body.

How much do you need to actively support your in- or outbreath so that the flow becomes deeper and longer?

What happens, if you neither draw in air actively with the inbreath, nor push with your abdominal muscles when you breathe out?

Does your breath become shallower or does it remain deep?

Try to expand your chest and tummy as far as possible with your breath.

Experiment:
- how much can you expand by actively supporting your breath?
- how much can you expand with your breath flowing freely?

Now allow your breath to return to its normal rhythm and depth.

Breathe out consciously a couple of times and let the inbreath happen by itself, that helps you to return to your own rhythm.

Allow your own breathing rhythm to flow with the intensity and frequency that is right for you.

Let it happen by itself, you don't have to actively support anything.

Observe your own rhythm for a while, flow with it, experience the waves inside you.

Change your position a little bit if you like, stretch and yawn and sigh.

Now, let's talk about our observations:
- what changes did you notice in your body when you breathed faster or slower?
- did any of you quite like the faster or slower breathing rhythm?
- could you become aware of the difference between actively supporting in- or outbreath and letting your breath flow freely?
- who did hyperventilate (get dizzy, get too much oxygen) during the fast or the slow breathing? Do you know what went wrong? [Breathing too deeply in the fast phase, or not slowly enough in the deep phase; now, in the relaxed situation the body does not need such an intensive breathing.]
- has your own rhythm changed in the course of the exercise? Was it deeper or shallower, faster or slower at the end compared to the beginning?
- what else did you notice when you experimented with your breathing?

EXERCISE
Breathing awareness
2

SEEING PATTERNS

Position: sit or lie down comfortably, as you prefer; change your position bit by bit until you feel really good about the way you are sitting or lying.

Aims:

○ Greater awareness of one's own rhythm
○ Experimentation with nuances of different rhythms
○ Comparing rhythms with the other participants and experiencing individual differences

○ Allowing the antenatal teacher to see the individual breathing patterns more clearly, so that she can build on their strengths and attend to their weaknesses.

Take your time.

Now, concentrate on your breathing.

Feel its flow.

Let a graphic image of your breath originate in your mind.

Breathe along its curves.

How do you see your breath?
  – as waves, as a zig-zag curve, as an infinite circle?

What does your picture look like?

Experiment a little with your breath and change the picture accordingly.

Now imagine a different picture and try to breathe according to this representation.

Take your time.

Try out different breathing patterns and images.

Which do you like?

Which don't suit you?

Feel which patterns flow easily and which need effort.

Now allow your breathing to return to the rhythm which comes by itself, without any effort, and find a graphic image for *your* rhythm.

Now, stretch and move about a bit, and come back to the group.

Draw the graph picture on the paper provided.

EXERCISE
Breathing awareness
3

CONTINUOUS BREATHING

Position: sit or lie down; take your time about getting comfortable.

Aims:

○ To experience the negative effect of holding a pause for too long
○ To become more aware of what rhythms suit everybody individually

Now, concentrate on your breathing again.

Feel its flow.

Follow the movements of your body while you are breathing in and out.

Observe what is happening at the moment when you are neither breathing in nor out: is there a pause after the in- or outbreath? Or is there a continuous flow without a pause?

Experiment a little with your breathing.

Let there be a pause after the inbreath; try pauses of different length.

How do you experience the pauses following the inbreath?

What is happening in your body?

How long can you pause without feeling uneasy?

Let your breathing return to your normal rhythm again.

Now, experiment with pauses following the outbreath.

How do you experience those?

What is happening in your body?

How long can you pause without feeling uneasy?

Now, let your breathing return to the rhythm that comes by itself. If you feel a bit dizzy, cup your mouth and nose with your hands and breathe in your own outbreath for a while.

Now let your breath flow again without any effort.

Feel the flow of your breath and try to breathe for a while without pausing.

Imagine a circle or a wave which you follow with your breath, a flowing transition from inbreath to outbreath.

Maybe the image of waves on a beach might help you: their relentless forming and ebbing.

Try to let it happen.

If it is too fast for you, breathe more slowly; find your own speed.

If you get too much oxygen, regulate the intensity of your breath.

Breathe as shallowly or as deeply as your body needs, as slowly and as lightly as you want, in and out without pausing.

Stay acutely aware of your breathing and regulate speed and intensity as you need it.

And now allow your breathing to change if it wants to.

Pause if your body needs to.

Let your own rhythm flow again.

Now, stretch and yawn, and sigh, and come back to the group.

Discussion:
 – what did you experience?
 – what did you observe?
 – how do you feel now?

EXERCISE
Breathing awareness
4

WALKING IN A CIRCLE

The participants should do at least one circle in each variation, in small rooms they could walk two circles.

With every new suggestion invite them to become aware of whether there is something changing in their breathing and what is happening as a response in their body (hands tightening, turning outwards or inwards etc.).

The sequence of the variation is arranged to increase the stress gradually.

Instructions:

Walk in a circle until your breathing gets into a natural flow.

Walk on the tips of your toes. Become aware of the change in your breathing.

Walk on your heels, become aware of the change in your breathing.

Walk on the outer edges of your feet. Become aware of the change of the breath etc.

Walk on the inner edges of the feet. Become aware of the change in your breathing.

Squat and walk squatting. Become aware of the change in your breathing.

EXERCISE
Breathing sounds 1

BREATHING WITH SOUND

Position: sitting on a chair, legs spread apart, lean forward onto a table. Or sitting on a folded blanket on the floor leaning forwards onto your hands. The tummy should be allowed to hang loose, without the back arched. Feet or legs should be placed firmly on the floor.

Aims:

 ○ Allows breath to flow deeper
 ○ Encourages participants to experiment with sounds, audible sighs and groans in public

    ○ Encourages participants to find their own sound
    ○ Encourages participants to make their own sounds however ill-fitting they may be.

Breathe deeply.

Allow your back to expand and widen with each inbreath.

Allow your tummy to relax and widen with each outbreath.

Place one hand on your tummy and feel how it softens with the outbreath. Don't use your abdominal muscles to force out more air than necessary.

[Ask whether everybody can do the exercise or if anyone has difficulties with it so far and deal with them before you continue.]

Allow a sound to come with each outbreath: groan, sigh, 'haah', 'huuh', 'hoo', 'haoum', for only as long as your outbreath flows: don't tense your abdominal muscles. Don't force any sound.

Try different sounds on different levels; higher and lower notes, different vowels.

Share and discuss the observations in the group.

EXERCISE
Breathing sounds 2

'SOUNDING' IN THE CIRCLE

The group is sitting comfortably in a circle with everyone leaning slightly forward so that tummies can widen loosely.

Some tips and commentary to this exercise:

○ Offer a sound first and ask the group to tune in with it during the following outbreath and to vary it with their next outbreath
○ Check whether the group has understood the task as it is very disruptive if questions arise in the middle of the exercise. Make a clear arrangement that it is always the partner on the left (or the right) whose turn is next, so that everybody knows when they are due to introduce their sound
○ Most participants find it easier to make a sound in public if this is described as singing or toning rather than groaning
○ The participants get a chance to find their own sound by copying the sounds of others (sounds they might not have thought of), and by having to vary them additionally
○ Every participant can make her/his sound as loudly or quietly as she/he likes. It is often useful to add a second round, or to repeat the exercise later on, as most people allow themselves to make more sound second time round
○ Disharmony is natural and all right. If ten or more people make spontaneous sounds, this does not need to sound

harmonious. This is important practice for the participants in sticking to their own sound despite the disharmony – and even to become louder rather than quieter. It is also a good experience to allow oneself one's own sound rather than succumbing to group pressure

○ Remind the participants not to push out excess air and sound with their abdominal muscles. The idea of the exercise is not to hold the sound for as long as possible, but to loosen the breath and to experiment with different sounds

○ Remind participants to explore deep and open sounds 'a', 'o', 'u' but to experiment also with 'e' and 'i', to experience the effect of the various sounds on them. Under stress we often tend to make tightly squeezed whimpering sounds that don't release any tension. So, encourage participants to make open and deep sounds if that feels right to them

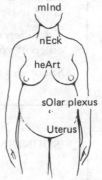

○ It will help if you can demonstrate the difference between open and tight sounds

○ In some groups it is important to encourage participants now and then (during the round without interrupting it) to allow louder sounds, to open their mouth and throat more

○ A valuable hint for the birth partner is to watch out for tight sounds, or sounds made with an inbreath. This indicates that the woman wants to vocalize and he can then help her to make open sounds with the outbreath, possibly by making them himself

Everybody in turn makes their own sound, any vowel and tone they choose, while breathing out. The others in the group tune in. With the next outbreath the same person makes his/her sound again and this time each of the other participants makes his or her complementary sound to this first sound. It can be higher or lower using the same vowel, or the same note but using a different vowel.

Thus, the group creates a rich chord of different sounds which resonate with the sound of one particular person.

With the next outbreath the next person in the circle introduces her/his sound. The group tunes in, and with the next outbreath everybody varies the given sound etc. This continues until everyone in the circle has had their turn.

EXERCISE
Breathing sounds 3

ALTERNATIVE 'SOUNDING'

As a group find a joint breathing rhythm, possibly by conducting it with your hands (see page 112).

Suggest to the participants to make a sound with each outbreath and encourage different sounds, vowels and tones. As with the exercise above it is important for participants to accept the disharmony and practise sticking to their own sound.

Another way of introducing the theme of sounds in labour, is to play a tape recording of 'labour noises': heavy breathing, groans, sounds, sighs, moans, nonsense babbling. Ask participants to listen to it with closed eyes. This often provides a more honest and vivid account of the reality of labour than pictures or slides can present.

Pair exercises

In some groups it is beneficial if the woman starts off as the 'partner'. She is often more sensitive and the exercises become more effective that way as she then gives her partner ideas on how she would like things done.

PAIR EXERCISE 1

FOLLOWING THE MOVEMENT OF THE BREATH

The partner is sitting on the floor, leaning his back against the wall. The woman is sitting in his lap, leaning her back against him. He embraces her with his arms and places his hands on both sides of her tummy.

The woman tries to reach his hands with her breath, so that he feels the movements of her breathing beneath his hands.

Both watch the rhythm of the woman's breathing

Then the partner puts his hands on the sides of her chest

The woman tries to reach his hands with her breath, so that he feels the movements of her breathing beneath his hands. They compare the rhythm of the breathing: then and now?

The partner places his hands just below the collar bones (effectively, the upper parts of the lungs).

The woman tries again to reach his hands with her breath so that he feels the movement of her breathing beneath his hands.

They compare the rhythm of her breathing: then and now?

The partner places his hands again on the side of the chest . . . etc.

The woman lets her breath travel down, and finishes with deep belly-breathing.

For women who would like to breathe deeper but cannot 'reach' their belly, then suggest deep, relaxed breathing with sounds or try the following pair exercise.

Now, change roles.

PAIR EXERCISE 2

VARIATION

The partner is sitting behind the woman, so that he can touch her back easily (both on the floor or on chairs, the woman leaning over the back of the chair).

The partner places his hands on her waist (kidney area). She tries to reach his hands with her breath. Both watch the woman's breathing rhythm.

The partner puts his hands on the sides of her chest. She tries to reach his hands with her breath.

They compare the breathing rhythm: then, and now?

The partner places both hands below the collar bones (he embraces her without pressure). She tries to reach his hands with her breath. They compare the breathing rhythm: then, and now?

Again, the hands and the breath wander down, to finish with deep breathing.

PAIR EXERCISE 3

INVITING THE BREATH TO FLOW DEEPER

In doing these exercises there is the danger that people 'learn' to produce a breathing unnatural to them, stressing the inbreath to reach the hands. Point out that the aim is not to become 'master of the deepest breath'.

Aim:

○ To become aware and get to know one's own breathing rhythm and depths

○ To experience what feels good and what doesn't
○ To train the partner in breathing awareness (the partner should not correct the pattern, but learn to become aware of the breathing needs and rhythm of his partner)
○ To let the breath flow deeply, without effort.

The woman is lying or sitting comfortably and relaxedly. The breath flows freely.

The partner watches the depth of the breath and its movement. He puts his hands where he sees the strongest movement. After some breaths he moves his hands a couple of inches down (on the chest, back or tummy, depending on the place the woman is breathing into).

The woman tries to reach this place with her breath.

The partner watches: is the breath still flowing freely? If it is, he can move his hands downwards another inch. If he becomes aware that his partner is sucking in air or needs to push to reach his hands, he then places them a little bit higher again.

Now change roles.

Group discussion:
  – how was this exercise for everybody?
  – where were the difficulties?
  – which breathing felt most natural?

PAIR EXERCISE 4

BREATHING AWARENESS AND ATTUNING

The partner is sitting on a chair; the woman is kneeling in front of him, putting the upper part of her body in his lap (her back should be round, the knees supported by a cushion or blanket, the pelvis flexible).

This exercise is also possible in the following position: The partner is sitting comfortably on the floor with a cushion, his back leaning against the wall. The woman is sitting between his legs, leaning back against him. Or you could just suggest that the couples find a position that is comfortable to both of them in which they have maximal body contact without impeding each other.

Aim:

○ Attuning in to the partner
○ Feeling which flows most easily. What comes naturally, what needs an effort? When guiding or following the partner?
○ Trying out the rhythms suggested for the different stages of labour. (see page 109).

The partner embraces her with his arms, so that he can feel as much as possible of her without impeding her.

The woman tries all the different breathing rhythms she can think of in irregular sequence and length.

The man tries to tune his rhythm into hers, so that they are breathing together with the woman 'leading'.

Now, change roles.

PAIR EXERCISE 5

RESPONDING TO PRESSURE

The aim of the exercise is not to find the right breathing for labour, but to learn to become aware of what our bodies do spontaneously and to let ourselves know whether or not we are comfortable with it.

The partner sits on the floor leaning comfortably against the wall.

The woman sits well back between his legs (possibly on a folded blanket to sit a bit higher), and leans against his chest.

The partner puts his arms around the woman's tummy with his hands overlapping just below her navel.

The woman encourages the partner to gently and gradually pull the tummy inwards towards himself.

They give feedback to each other on how it feels.

Most partners fear they could be doing harm and are relieved to hear the woman say that it does not hurt.

The pulling in of the tummy is a simulation of what the uterus does when contracting during labour.

The woman explores what happens to her breathing as her partner gives her a simulated contraction:
- does she spontaneously breathe away from the pressure, breathing more lightly and shallowly?
- does she spontaneously breathe deeper into her tummy to meet the pressure?

The woman can observe clearly what her own tendency is.

The woman and partner now try out the opposite of what she did spontaneously and note how it feels. They might be surprised that it feels better; or know for sure that this is not what they are comfortable with.

Although this is a valuable observation and a good exercise in awareness, they should not draw the conclusion that this is what their breathing should be like in labour.

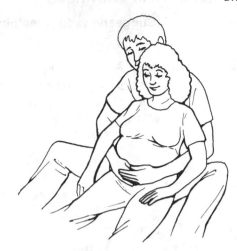

BREATHING IN LABOUR

Breathing during a contraction

We should try to allow our body to breathe as intensively as it needs to at all times. However, because we tend to interfere with our breathing in situations of fear, stress and pain some guidelines on breathing might be useful.

The following points may not suit every teacher or every class. They are included however, as they may be useful for participants who have very little breathing awareness and/or expect to 'learn' breathing from the antenatal teacher. They fulfil this need whilst at the same time encouraging more self-awareness.

Start every contraction with an outbreath

The conventional rule of greeting the contraction with an inbreath only intensifies the tendency to take a deep breath and to hold it until the pain goes away. As contractions last longer than we can hold our breath this tendency is not very helpful in labour. Of course, if the labouring woman has just finished an outbreath when the next contraction sets in, she should let the inbreath stream into her as usual and then focus on the outbreath. The idea is 'to let yourself into the contraction' with the outbreath instead of fighting it.

Emphasize the outbreath throughout the contraction however shallow, deep, fast or slow your breathing

With the outbreath let go of any tension, let off steam, make room inside yourself. Because the outbreath is emphasized, it is slightly shorter than the inbreath, otherwise we would be pushing out too much air (see reference to hyperventilation page 93). The inbreath is slightly longer, as the breath is allowed to stream into the body rather than actively drawn in.

End each contraction with two deep breaths

With the first outbreath sigh and let go of any tension that has built up inside you during the contraction. With the second outbreath allow yourself to melt, to become soft and relaxed so that you can enjoy the interval between contractions.

Suggestions for breathing rhythms during first stage of labour

EXAMPLE 1   Deep continuous breathing with emphasized outbreath, possibly sighing or groaning with each outbreath: 'aaah', 'ooh', 'uuuh', 'haoum'. It is possible to breathe continuously deeply and slowly throughout labour, possibly getting gradually louder as labour gets more intense

breathing
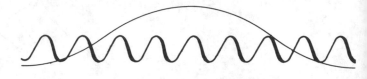

EXAMPLE 2   Some women find that their breathing becomes shallower and faster as the contraction gets more intense. (It is especially useful with this faster rhythm to demonstrate false breathing by actively drawing in air with each inbreath. This quickly leads to a sense of panic and to hyperventilation.)

breathing
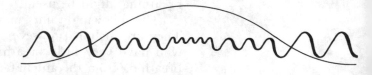

EXAMPLE 3   Some women find that their breathing becomes even deeper and slower as the contraction gets more intense.

breathing
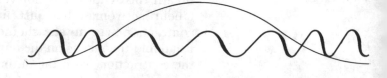

EXAMPLE 4   Some women remain continuously in deep breathing but adapt to the intensity of the contraction by allowing themselves to breathe faster and slower according to felt need.

breathing
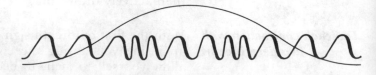

EXAMPLE 5   Another rhythm observed as occurring spontaneously in labours probably develops due to the overwhelming sensations that almost take your breath away, that almost makes you stop mid-breath. Using this tendency to stop mid-breath as a rhythm, one can climb over the intense sensations of the contraction. Every woman can (and while exploring in class) take one, two or three steps on either the inbreath or the outbreath or both, according to felt need.

breathing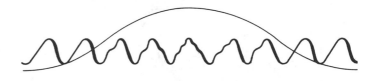

These rhythms are not to be learnt by heart and practised at home. The aim in introducing them in the classes is for the class participants to:

- ○ Explore different rhythms
- ○ Widen their range of breathing
- ○ Find out which rhythms suit them individually.

Most participants will spontaneously choose one or two rhythms that they feel comfortable with. Some participants will like all of them and want to practise them in real life, under the stress of, for example, climbing several flights of stairs. This will help them find the rhythms that suit them best. Others will find their own variation to some of the rhythms suggested, spontaneously, and feel comfortable with the adaptations.

Remind participants that whatever rhythms they choose in class, they should remain flexible and listen to their body's needs. What might suit them in the class environment, or as they climb upstairs, might not be the rhythm their body needs or wants in labour. This is why it is a good idea to increase the range of available rhythms women have and can fall back on.

In class try introducing the different rhythms by showing the breathing with your hands and arms.

The deeper the breathing the more you move your arms; the shallower the breathing, the smaller the movement is, until it is only the fingers that move up and down. As the arms/hands/fingers move up, the participants breathe in. As they move down the participants breathe out. Indicate the depth, rhythm and speed or slowness of the breathing with these movements. You can experiment with this in front of a mirror.

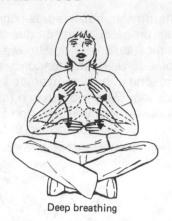

Deep breathing

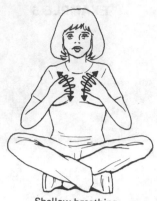

Shallow breathing

Sometimes there are teachers who want to teach a particular approach to breathing having learnt an entirely different technique for their own labours. When they use their hands to demonstrate a rhythm their bodies often 'betray' their minds. They may speak of letting the inbreath come by itself and of emphasizing the outbreath, yet their arms move actively and quite quickly upwards to indicate the inbreath, and lower themselves slowly to indicate the outbreath. Be careful of giving double messages this way in class.

It is important for participants to overcome any ideas of 'right' or 'wrong' breathing, and to stress that there is no 'ideal' (such as breathing as deeply as possible, or into the chest, or on the count of seven). Were they to regard only a smooth, flowing, deep breathing as ideal, for example, and then find themselves spontaneously doing the opposite in labour – breathing shallowly or with sobs and steps – they would then think that they are doing something wrong, that they had 'failed'. If, on the other hand, they have experienced a wide range of rhythms beforehand, and learnt to accept and go along with these, they are more likely to accept themselves and to go along with their bodies' spontaneous rhythms during labour.

Sometimes one encounters participants who have already learnt a certain type of breathing somewhere else. They don't have to change their breathing if they are genuinely comfortable with this pattern and can, of course, bring it into their labour. However, it is still a good idea to encourage them to experiment with different rhythms; the body can then use whatever rhythm it needs at any given time.

While breathing patterns should not be imposed on anybody, teach only what you really believe in. It is your confidence that counts more than any rules or techniques. It is nevertheless valuable to try out the different rhythms (here and now as you are reading, and at other times, when you are climbing stairs or running for a bus); be open to experiment with your breathing.

When practising the rhythms in class, i.e. in a relatively un-stressed situation, the breathing should be kept light. Be careful not to demonstrate in a louder and more intense way than is appropriate to the here-and-now. Participants need to be able to see and hear what you mean, but explain that unless they keep their own breathing fairly light they won't be able to judge properly whether a particular rhythm feels comfortable to them or not.

Demonstrate the rhythms sitting comfortably in a circle, and then try them out in other positions. It is important not to suggest to participants that they lie down or sit back comfortably, as this would imply that good breathing *means* sitting back or lying down. Breathing can flow in any position, at any time. After they have tried out the rhythms in the position of their own choice, you can offer stress exercises or the stress sequence (see page 122) so that they can explore which of the rhythms suit them or arise spontaneously when their bodies are active.

Suggestions for breathing rhythms during transition

As contractions are usually very strong towards the end of first stage, and often also irregular and erratic, many labouring women find it difficult to maintain free flowing breathing during this time. Often, too, the midwife expects a breathing pattern which suppresses the urge to bear down, while the cervix isn't fully dilated. Nevertheless, many women are still able to maintain a deep flowing breathing all the way through labour. Some just sighed or groaned louder during transition.

EXAMPLE 1

A lot of women have the desire to breathe quite fast and shallowly. To prevent hyperventilation or panicking into ever faster and faster breathing, there are three rhythms to help women give in to their own need to breathe faster yet still to hold on to a firm rhythm.

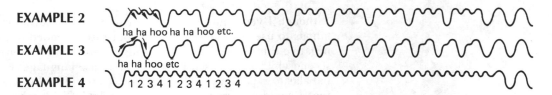

EXAMPLE 2 ha ha hoo ha ha hoo etc.

EXAMPLE 3 ha ha hoo etc

EXAMPLE 4 1 2 3 4 1 2 3 4 1 2 3 4

The last has no visual sign of rhythm but as a visual image which the woman can hold on to as she breathes:

> Imagine a birthday cake with four candles. Imagine showing your child *how* to blow out the candles. Don't actually blow them out, just blow *at* them, get them to flicker. Now blow at those four candles over and over again without pausing for a deep breath in between.

As it is better to avoid a deep breath in between, it is important to keep the 'hoo' of the first two shallow patterns short. To let go with the 'hoo' would mean a tendency to draw in a deep breath afterwards and to use that inbreath for holding it in and bearing down – an action not advisable in transition stage. Unless the cervix is completely dilated, any bearing down is a waste of energy, and undue pressure could cause the cervix to tear. Furthermore, the holding in of breath withholds the flow of oxygen to the baby.

However, if a woman becomes very tense by stopping herself from bearing down in transition, she is working against her own body. It can be argued she should go with her body's signals as long as she does not exhaust herself and as long as she does not hold her breath to bear down.

Quite often women find that nothing much helps at this transition stage. They keep themselves going and breathing with a wailing or pleading sing-song:

EXAMPLE 5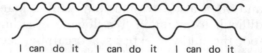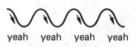

Encourage participants to think of rhythmic sentences, phrases or words that they would like to use in labour. You could mention Thomas the Tank Engine and his carriages: 'We're coming along, we're coming along'.

> One woman used 'O-pen o-pen o-pen' all through transition. When she talked about this at the class reunion, her husband was surprised "I thought at the time that you said pain-oh, pain-oh.

Women find it is much easier to let out their true feelings, and wail and moan: 'I can't, I can't' or 'No no no!' rather than sticking to positive suggestions.

> Although I very much wanted to, I was unable during my first labour to use positive suggestions, but rather tended to say negative things which I didn't really mean. So at the birth of my second child I expressed myself in nonsense language 'Kokeui babalasito raja dinale panina ta'. It was wonderfully relieving that I could express myself without anybody, including myself, giving it a negative label.

Suggestions for breathing rhythms in second stage of labour

Unfortunately, it is still common to recommend a 'breathing' pattern for second stage of holding one's breath and bearing down for as long as possible:

holding breath and pushing   holding breath and pushing

The myth of pushing as long and as hard as possible and its disadvantages

With this type of breathing-and-pushing rhythm, both baby and mother often end up exhausted, sometimes with the result that a forceps delivery becomes necessary. Those babies that are born within a few contractions with this type of pushing would have probably been born within a few contractions anyway, even if the mother hadn't pushed.

○ The woman bearing down this way does not get enough oxygen as she doesn't take in enough and holds her breath too long.
○ The uterus gets too little oxygen and ceases to work effectively
○ The baby gets too little oxygen and responds with a drop in the heart rate.

Additional to these factors which often 'necessitate' an obstetric intervention, this type of pushing has other disadvantages.

○ The woman is often pushing before she even feels the pushing urge, which makes the pushing subjectively more exhausting than if she could 'give in to' the urge.
○ With this type of prolonged pushing the throat and mouth, and with it the pelvic floor, get tightened which can lead to tearing or the necessity of an episiotomy.

The fact that a great many babies are born successfully *despite* these side-effects of the conventional management of second stage labour demonstrates how 'hardy' babies are and how our bodies cope with adverse circumstances. But it should not be used as an excuse to continue with this method.

Focusing on breathing rather than pushing in second stage eases the stress for mothers and babies, which is reason enough to give up the conventional method. Babies can be born successfully without any additional pushing, and this is proven by the numerous women who: have given birth on the way to hospital or while waiting for the midwife and desperately *not* pushing; by women who, for medical reason, are not allowed to push; and by women who try the gentle approach to second stage in particular and to childbirth as a whole.

Nevertheless it may be useful to ask the men in the group to adopt the 'classical' bearing-down position and, guiding them through a 'normal' bearing-down type contraction, urge them to 'push-push-push, and a little longer' etc. Once such a 'bearing-down' contraction has been experienced partners may be much more likely to support their women through a contraction in second stage with the emphasis on breathing and opening, rather than on pushing.

There still prevails the ill founded belief we should hold our breath when doing something strenuous. (Observe yourself when lifting something heavy!) Yet if we observe weight lifters or masters of the martial arts they let go of air and sound while lifting or delivering the blow.

The pushing urge does not run parallel to the contraction

During a forceful outbreath the tummy muscles and the muscles alongside the spine become tightened so the person is stronger in doing whatever is required. Why then, one wonders, do so many midwives and obstetricians still encourage – if not force – women to hold their breath and to keep their mouth closed! Caldeyro Barcia's scientific work has now shown what women who were allowed to give birth their own way knew all along: that a contraction in second stage is not the same thing as a pushing urge; instead pushing urges *ride* the contraction:

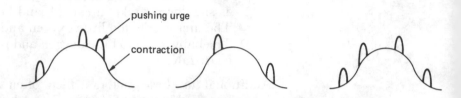

These pushing urges are convulsive and may last for only a few seconds. If the woman hasn't been pushing artificially already (thus missing the natural 'convulsion') she can't help but follow the urge and bear down. This bearing down lasts only for a few seconds, following which there may or may not be another urge soon after, although the contraction still goes on, irrespectively. Especially in the early part of second stage there are often a few contractions without any pushing urge at all.

Caldeyro Barcia also found out that holding one's breath longer than 6 seconds at any one time impeded the flow of oxygen. It is interesting that the 'convulsive' urges don't last longer than 4–5 seconds; Nature knows what she is doing. The woman should be encouraged to focus on providing oxygen to her hard-working body and to her baby, and on relaxing and opening herself (This is where the pelvic floor exercises become important (see page 139)). If there is no progress and the baby's head does not become any more visible (or feelable) inside the vagina a change of position is best (see page 150). Changing into an upright position, may suddenly bring on the urge to push, as the baby's head is now pressing down with the weight of gravity. For some women the opposite is true: they feel the pushing urge for the first time or more strongly once they allow themselves (or are encouraged) to lie down. It is the baby's head, then pressing on the back passage, which can trigger the sensation of wanting to push.

I remained upright with both my labours. I had a few pushing urges with each second stage contraction during the first birth and no pushing urge whatsoever during the second birth. But then the second baby was two pounds heavier than the first one and it is possible that my pelvic floor just needed that extra time and gentleness to stretch around this big baby. I am sure that had I pushed, without the invitation of my body to do so, I would have torn or needed an episiotomy.

With the following four rhythms the woman can work with, instead of against, her body. At the beginning of each contraction she breathes out, lets herself into the contraction, allows the contraction to come, to become stronger, and then follows the pushing urge if and when she feels it.

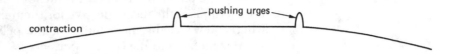

Assuming there is a contraction with pushing urges at these times, the breathing rhythm could then be charted as follows:

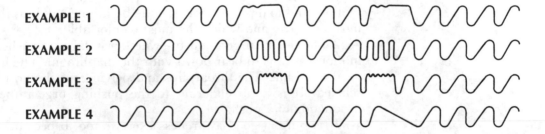

1 As the woman feels the pushing urge she breathes in-out-in-out quickly (like a diver before entering the water) to pump herself full of oxygen. The body can receive more oxygen this way than with one deep inbreath. Then, she just bears down holding her breath as long as she feels the pushing urge. The woman can close her mouth, but should make sure the lips, jaws and throat remain relaxed and soft. It is possible not to let any air out while bearing down despite an open mouth and throat. Try it!)

2 The woman breathes deeply continuously through the contraction. Her breathing gets faster and more intense as she bears down with the pushing urge. It is possible to bear down effectively while continuing a deep breathing.

3 As she feels the pushing urge, the woman breathes lightly and shallowly while at the same time bearing down. Mouth and throat can remain wide open and relaxed. To breathe lightly and shallowly does not prevent or inhibit bearing down, despite contrary beliefs.

4 As she bears down with the urge, the woman breathes out very slowly as if downwards and out through her vagina.

In class encourage participants to place the palm of their hands on their pelvic floor (men have the same muscles and feel a similar effect). Ask them to repeat the pelvic floor exercise where they 'take the lift into several floors' up, and down again. Once they get to the 'ground floor' ask them to go to the 'basement'. Now, in order to go to the 'basement' – to get the pelvic floor to bulge slightly outwards – one can either hold one's breath and bear down gently, or continue breathing deeply, or do shallow breathing, or let the breath out very gradually, while bearing down gently as in the rhythms above. Encourage participants to try all the four methods and to feel which of the methods is the most effective for them personally; it will be the one where they feel the most bulge of the pelvic floor with their hand.

If somebody in the class experiences absolutely no bulge, have her (or him) breathe into an empty, clean bottle while placing her hand on her pelvic floor. As soon as her breath hits the bottom of the bottle, a pelvic floor bulge will appear against her hand. She can then widen her pelvic floor without the help of the bottle.

Experimenting with pushing without strain

Suggest to the class participants to try out the different breathing rhythms for second stage whenever they go to the toilet to pass a motion, and to discover which of the breathing rhythms they find the most effective, and which the most comfortable.

To follow the urge to push – whether in labour or when passing a motion – means to bear down with the diaphragm. The lungs do not need to be full. The throat, lips and pelvic floor should be open and relaxed. It is a surrendering to the pushing urge rather than the production of a push.

It is quite a good awareness exercise too to become sensitive to when one actually wants to pass a motion. Can you wait for the pushing urge or do you go to the toilet and begin 'straining' because you 'think' you have to pass a motion? Or because the clock tells you to? There is a parallel here to the hospital birth where the midwife wants the baby to be born within a certain time once the cervix is dilated. To experience the satisfaction of passing a motion in its own time can give you the strength to want to give birth to your baby in its own time too. Once women have practised and experienced the possibility of bearing down without holding their breath and straining they will be much more able to do so in labour. Again and again I find that midwives and doctors are willing to go along with a woman's or couple's 'strange' wishes as long as labour progresses and the baby is fine. The baby is much more likely to be fine if it gets all the oxygen it needs. Labour is much more likely to progress if the woman is able to loosen up, be open and *let* the baby out.

Stress exercises

Exercises through which not only breathing rhythms but also one's attitudes and responses to stress/pain can be explored.

**EXERCISE
Stress 1**

KNEELING

Duration: 1–2 min.

Position: kneel on the floor, heels together, knees as far apart as possible.

Lean forward, lowering yourself with your hands, until your left or right ear is lying on the floor, while your buttocks are resting on your heels.

Some women and men find the stretching of the thighs very painful. Others enjoy it. Just as it is with early contractions: some feel them as pleasant sensations, for others they hurt.

**EXERCISE
Stress 2**

LEG ROLLING

With this exercise participants simulate the work of the contraction: the physical labour, the exhaustion, but also the climax as the contraction increases and decreases in intensity.

Duration: 1–2 min.

Position: sit on the floor. Legs straight, spread as far apart as possible.

Lean backwards onto your hands. Begin to roll your feet – always emphasizing the outwards movement to prevent the legs from gliding together.

Keep rolling – take the support of your arms away, sitting upright.

Keep rolling – stretch your arms out sideways.

Keep rolling – stretch your arms out above your head.

Keep rolling – stretch your arms out sideways.

Keep rolling – lower your arms and remain sitting upright.

Keep rolling – lean back onto your hands.

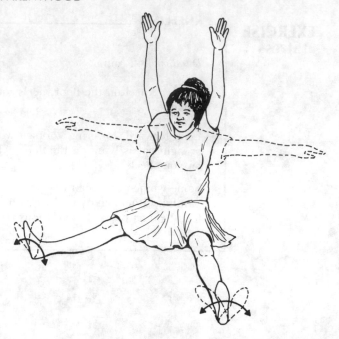

The following three stress exercises are quite strenuous if done correctly. As they 'work' the thigh muscles they do not affect uterus or pelvic floor adversely. It is very easy to cheat with these exercises or to stop whenever the body does not want to take any more stress.

**EXERCISE
Stress 3**

RIDER'S POSITION

Duration: 1–2 min.

Position: Standing, feet shoulder-width apart.

Bend your knees, the soles of the feet staying firmly on the floor.

Bend your knees further, as if on horseback, until the tension in your thighs feels uncomfortable.

Don't lean forward; the back should be straight.

Bear the tension.

Breathe – don't fight.

Give in to the pain, find your own breathing rhythm.

Let your pelvis circle; move with the pain.

After a while, stretch your legs, move and loosen them.

Breathe deeply twice, let go of any tension.

**EXERCISE
Stress 4**

RIDER'S POSITION: VARIATION

A more challenging version of the 'Rider's Position' can be achieved if the participants first squat and then from the squatting position move into the rider's position.

**EXERCISE
Stress 5**

RIDER'S POSITION: AS A PAIR EXERCISE

Duration: $1\frac{1}{2}$ min.

Stand opposite each other holding hands with arms comfortably outstretched.

Together, descend into a squatting position, still holding hands.

If necessary, adjust your distance to one another.

Neither of you should hang onto the other; instead maintain your own firm stand or, rather, squat.

Find a mutual long deep breathing rhythm.

Come up together into the rider's position, keeping your backs straight, holding hands without clinging and maintaining eye contact.

Breathe together.

Allow yourselves to make sounds – groans and sighs – together and for each other.

Depending on what you prefer, both make a sound with the outbreath in unison. Or, as one of you breathes in, the other one breathes out and vice-versa, so that one of you is always making a sound. A see-saw of sighs, groans. This way tension gets expressed continuously even as you breathe in.

Then both stand upright again, loosen your legs, move about a bit.

**EXERCISE
Stress 6**

RIDER'S POSITION: AT THE WALL

This is an extremely strenuous way of sitting which reminds most women, who have already given birth, of labour.

Ask the partners to do it first so that they experience the intense sensation and are able to concentrate on their own breathing without worrying how their women are coping. Then ask the women to do it, working with their breathing, sighs and groans, their partners standing by and ready to give them support, if it should get too much.

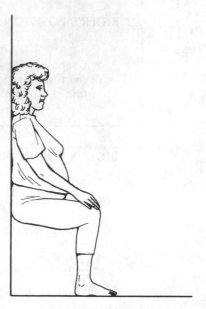

Stand, feet apart, about one foot away from the wall. Lean against the wall, until comfortable, then bending your knees, let your back glide down the wall, until your thighs are parallel to the floor. Keep this position for $1-1\frac{1}{2}$ min. until the simulated contraction is over, then come up again. (If you can, but listen to your body, it may be better to go down onto the floor and come up from there on hands and knees.)

EXERCISE
Stress 7

STRESS SEQUENCE

This sequence contains five simulated contractions. Let each simulated contraction last for $1-1\frac{1}{2}$ minutes, perhaps increasing the time to $1\frac{1}{2}-2$ minutes when you repeat the sequence at a later session. Give the participants 2–3 minutes' break between the simulated contractions to recover. Talk them through the whole sequence, reminding them to breathe out, to let go, to let-off steam, to make sounds, to loosen their pelvises and pelvic floors and anything else that you see them tensing up during the simulations. Give them some prompting during the 'breaks' reminding them to relax, to change position, to loosen up, to be grateful for each contraction that brings them closer to the birth of their child, and to look forward to the next strong and effective one. Remind them that the next 'contraction' will come in 40 or 20 seconds, whenever you intend it, so that they will be mentally prepared. Don't tell the participants that the sequence contains five simulated contractions, as, in real labour, they won't know how many more contractions there will be.

Best done just after the exercise To Open and to Accept Help (see p. 000), as the loins are softened and the pain felt in the following sequence is more intense.

Walking in a Circle (see page 102):	Labour begins, slight discomfort
Kneeling, knees apart, buttocks on heels, left or right ear on the floor:	Contractions get stronger but not everybody feels pain yet
Leg Rolling (see page 138):	Contractions experienced as labour, as work, as exhausting, though not necessarily as painful
Rider's Position (from standing), (see page 120):	Contractions get stronger still, most people will feel the stress and the 'pain'
Rider's Position (from squatting) (see page 121):	Contractions get stronger still
Rider's Position against the Wall (see page 121):	Contractions are really strong now; this is effective, good, established labour.

**EXERCISE
Stress 8**

TICKLING

Duration: 1–2 min.

Position: The woman adopts a position where she feels most in contact with herself, protected, and strong.

Aim:

○ To tolerate irritating sensations, without fighting them or tensing up against them.
○ To stay calm whatever happens, working with breathing and sound.

The woman concentrates on a deep, relaxed breathing and stays with herself and her relaxation.

The partner then starts tickling her and so gives an irritating stimulus (labour).

The woman tries to concentrate and stay relaxed by breathing.

She tries different breathing rhythms to find out which helps her most. She doesn't let herself become distracted.

After 1 min: no more tickling; end of simulated contraction.

The woman takes two deep breaths, lets go of accumulated tension, moves, changer her position.
  – which rhythm comes spontaneously?
  – which rhythm is particularly helpful for you in staying with yourself?

DRESS REHEARSAL FOR BIRTH

This is just one model for a dress rehearsal; you can mix and match any breathing and positions that you teach. Make it quite clear to the participants that they don't have to use any of the combinations or the sequence, but that in their labours they will find their own combinations and sequences. Yet also point out that they don't have to be original either. If they want to use any of those combinations and feel happy with it at the time, that is fine. Be aware that if you hand out sheets with the main points for each stage of labour the participants could cling to it and refer to it rather than listening to their own bodies.

First stage of labour

Repeat briefly all the main points: signs of start of labour, routine procedures in hospital or at home, positions, tips, either by eliciting them or listing them yourself.

Duration	Position	Breathing	Interaction
$1\frac{1}{2}$ min.	Standing, leaning on wall, or on the partner	Deep slow continuous breathing.	Partner strokes with each outbreath along the arms, back, neck, etc. to emphasize the outbreath (see page 146).
$1\frac{1}{2}$ min.	Kneeling, leaning forward onto the bed, a chair, partner's lap, or pile of pillows.	Deep breathing with irregular, fast breaths in between.	Partner uses touch relaxation, slight pressure with each 'regular' outbreath to guide her back to her own original breathing rhythm (see page 145).
$1\frac{1}{2}$ min.	Lying on one side.	Gradually breathing more shallowly and quickly towards the height of contraction. Breathing deeper and more slowly again as the contraction fades away.	Partner gives a back massage applying counterpressure to where the baby's head presses against the spine (see page 147).
$1\frac{1}{2}$ min.	'Rider's position', hanging onto a frame or onto partner's shoulders.	Breathing with steps in and out.	Focus on relaxation of the pelvis floor, letting go, being open.

Duration	Position	Breathing	Interaction
1½ min.	Any position liked.	Deep, slow breathing getting even slower and deeper towards the height of contraction, returning to normal deep slow breathing as contraction recedes.	Express a wish to your partner for this contraction: 'Leave me alone this time;' 'Hold me tight' 'Stroke my . . .' 'Massage my . . .'.
1½ min.	Standing, with partner close behind.	Own breathing rhythm	Do a pelvic swing together (see page 138).
1½ min.	Any standing or kneeling position where your pelvis is free to move. Ask your partner for support if you want it.	Own breathing rhythm	Move, circle rotate pelvis freely (see page 134).
1½ min.	Any position liked.	Own breathing.	Move pelvis back and forth in tune with breathing: inbreath = pelvis tilted backwards; outbreath = pelvis tilted forward.

Transition

Repeat briefly the main points by eliciting or listing: irregularity of contractions; physical side-effects, wanting to give up, etc; positions; tips.

Duration	Position	Breathing	Interaction
1½ min.	Kneeling, head and chest lower than hips, moving trunk up and down as needed.	Talking, murmuring, wailing, praying, under one's breath.	
1½ min.	Lying on one side.	Using 'ha ha hoo' breathing, the rhythm of the four birthday candles, or any other light rhythm that feels right.	Massaging tummy with light strokes.
1½ min.	Tickling as stimulation of contraction (see page 123). Any position in which the woman feels she can cope with the disturbance.	Any breathing that helps to be with oneself.	Partner tickles, irritates, as best as he can.

Second stage of labour

Repeat briefly main points: to breathe, to open up, to let go, to keep the pelvis loose, to relax the pelvic floor.

Duration	Position	Breathing	Interaction
$1\frac{1}{2}$ min.	Half-sitting, pelvis flat on the mattress, upper part of the body rounded and supported by cushions or partner.	Guiding through a contraction, prompting with three pushing urges, asking woman to hold her breath for 5 s and to widen her pelvic floor.	Partner can sit behind woman, helping her into a semi-upright position, or sit next to her supporting her round the shoulders.
$1\frac{1}{2}$ min.	On all-fours, pelvis loose and flexible, top part of the body more or less raised.	Deep breathing, widening of pelvic floor as woman breathes shallowly and quickly for a few seconds as a response to the prompting of three pushing urges.	
$1\frac{1}{2}$ min.	Semi-squatting, supported by one or two people.	Deep, continuous, breathing. Responding to the prompting of three pushing urges while continuing to breathe deeply.	
$1\frac{1}{2}$ min	Kneeling, hanging on to partner or frame.	Deep breathing, letting the breath out very slowly with each prompted pushing urge.	

EXERCISES TO DO AT HOME

BREATHING: HOMEWORK

One homework task per session will feel about right. Tasks for homework can be combined or altered to suit your course structure. Participants are usually very keen to explore the various suggestions especially as they do not demand a particular time of day to be set aside or involve exercises that need a mat or special clothing etc. All that is required is that the participants become more aware of their body in everyday life – which is arguably the best preparation for childbirth.

Some suitable tasks:

1. Become aware of and observe your own breathing rhythm in different situations: during work, while walking, during a conversation, while watching TV, as you are about to fall asleep, while climbing several flights of stairs, while making love, during an internal examination, when you are tense or excited about something . . . anytime.
2. Become aware when you are actively helping your breath – drawing in air, forcing out more air than necessary – and allow your breathing consciously to flow freely.
3. Allow your breath to gradually flow more freely and deeply in all the above-mentioned situations, whenever you become aware of it.
4. Use the rules for breathing during a contraction for every stress situation in everyday life. As you become aware of the stress, breathe out consciously, let go of unnecessary tension and allow a free-flowing breath throughout. Become aware when the stress situation is over: breathe deeply two or three times and let go of any remaining tension with the outbreath.
5. Try out the breathing rhythms for the first stage of labour in strenuous everyday situations (like climbing several flights of stairs) or when you are in pain (headache, toothache etc.).
6. Think about phrases or words that you would like to use in labour (especially transition) and mumble them now and then under your breath.
7. Try the various breathing rhythms for bearing down when you pass a motion.

18 Body awareness and keep-fit exercises

REFLECTIONS What is the role of keep-fit exercises for you? Do you do any regularly? Do you do any in your classes? Did you do any while you were pregnant?

No element of antenatal teaching should be overvalued. Just as knowledge about the birth process, or good nutrition cannot produce a good birth, neither can keep-fit exercises. We should not give the impression in class that whoever practises these exercises regularly, can do them well and is physically fit, will have an easy labour. Although keep-fit exercises will not guarantee an easy labour, they are, nevertheless, of value. Keep-fit exercises are more than a strengthening of certain muscles: with exercise difference parts of the body are mobilized, blood flow is increased, particular parts of the body get warmer, and we become more aware of them. Exercises involving the whole body, particularly, serve to help the experience of one's body as a unity: its strength and its wholeness, as well as its tension, weakness and pain. Furthermore, with increased blood flow the tension can be released, as waste products get flushed out. Thus, keep-fit exercises in birth preparation classes can play different roles:

○ Strengthening and/or loosening certain parts of the body
○ Releasing tension
○ Increasing body self-awareness
○ Increasing tolerance thresholds

The physical exercises can be exploited differently, depending on which words you introduce and accompany them with. The physical processes accompanying exercise will happen regardless; what is less automatic and will need prompting is the self-awareness and tolerance thresholds. Focus the participants' awareness on these asking what they can feel in their body and how their breathing reacts at the various stages of the exercise.

Offer only as much keep-fit or body awareness exercises as you yourself enjoy; don't do anything just because you think you ought to.

When to use keep-fit/body awareness exercises

○ At the beginning of a session to loosen up and tune in
○ During the session to demonstrate a certain point or as a break after an intense discussion
○ To round the session off at the end.

In the course of a class you can add physical exercises with a different aim to each new session.

EXAMPLE

Session 1 onwards:	To loosen up, not only physically but with one another also. Exercises that prevent and combat back pain, varicose veins, cramps etc.
Session 2 onwards:	Experiencing the body as a whole. Becoming aware of one's breathing. Exercises to loosen pelvis and pelvic floor.
Session 3 onwards:	Combining body and breathing awareness with gymnastics. How do the parts of the body feel, before and after? What happens with the breathing?
Session 4 onwards:	Introducing stress exercises. Exploring the individual pain threshold – which breathing is useful?

Choose from the following exercises what you yourself enjoy doing and what seems to suit you and your class. You can vary, alter and supplement the exercises to meet your requirements. Of course, you can also offer totally different exercises, for example, if you have experience with yoga, Alexander technique etc. Offer whatever fits *your* aims that *you* have for your classes.

The exercises are also useful to sensitize the participants to the messages their bodies send them. With some of the more painful stretching exercises, such as squatting for example, the participants can become aware of their different responses to stress, and to pain: Wanting to fight it. Wanting to give in to it or recognizing it as a valuable message from the body that they have gone too far.

Exercises for fitness and body awareness

EXERCISES

TEN EXERCISES DONE STANDING

Participants stand with their feet about one hand's width apart. This is about the width of the pubic rami. The width between the ischial tuberosities varies individually. As this is the space the baby has to pass through it is a good exercise in body awareness for pregnant women to explore their individual width. If the feet stand too far apart or too close together then too much strain is put on the hip joints. It is interesting that there is a correlation between the width of the pubic rami, one's shoesize and the width of one's hand. Encourage participants to explore their own individual standing position where they are comfortable.

1 Stand, feet about a hand's breadth apart. Loosen your knees so that they are slightly bent. Bounce softly until you find the right position.

Your spine is resting on your pelvis; don't arch your back. Tilt your pelvis forward and back until you find a good position.

Let shoulders and arms hang loose.

Now move your head slowly, looking over your left shoulder then over your right shoulder.

Tilt your head to one side, then the other. Let your earlobes touch your shoulder.

Thrust your head upwards towards the ceiling.

Draw your shoulders up (inbreath), and let them drop (outbreath).

Circle your shoulders (inbreath: backwards/outbreath: forwards).

Move your shoulders forwards and backwards (moving backwards on the inbreath and forwards on the outbreath).

Similar to breaststroke. Bring your arms from the sides to the front of the chest, let your back and shoulders become round, while you are breathing in; move your hands forward and then to the sides, while you are breathing out.

Now, on the inbreath raise your arms slowly above your head.

On the outbreath, let them slowly sink down to your side.
On the inbreath, raise your arms slowly back above your head.

On the outbreath, let them drop down to your side, relaxed.

Do you observe the difference while breathing out?

2 Stretch your arms to the sides, bend your hands upward
= breathe in
let go = breathe out
Bend your fists downward = breathe in
let go = breathe out.

---

3 Indonesian Dance: Move all the joints of your arms, hands and fingers: how much movement is there in the joints?

---

4 Let your head hang down on your chest, feel the strain in the neck. Give in to the strain. Breathe. Relax your face, particularly around the mouth and the jaws.
Lift your head and then let it drop back. Give in to the uncomfortable strain, relax mouth- and jaw area. Breathe . . .

---

5 Starting from the head bend your spine slowly, vertebra after vertebra, until your whole body is hanging down. Then, starting with the lumbar vertebra, straighten your spine again. (If this is difficult, the partner can help by slowly stroking along the spine: the touched vertebra is bent or straightened.)

---

6 Massage your feet by shuffling them on the floor, particularly the upper side of the toes and feet.
Roll the inner and the outer edges of the feet.
Free exploration: what movements are possible? What else can we do with our feet on the ground besides walking or standing?

---

7 Shift your weight on to one leg. Lift the other one.
Move the joints of the leg and the foot without losing your balance: bend, circle, stretch. What is happening with your breathing? If necessary participants can hold on to back of a chair or something similar.

---

8 Belly-dancing: Sway and circle your pelvis. Explore small, large and wide movements. Take care that the movements start from the pelvis: don't let your body or your legs circle; shoulders and knees shouldn't move.

Pelvis-centre:

When you are able to move your pelvis independently of your chest and knees, then you can let them swing with the pelvis or in the opposite direction.

---

9 Expand, stretch, conscious deep breathing.

10 Moving on the spot as you like it: slowly or fast; jump, shake, circle, dance.

Keep moving, don't stop, don't think.

Just move somehow.

Use all parts of your body, all your joints, even those – and particularly those – which you don't use much normally.

Follow your own body.

Feel how your body wants to move, feel which movements are uncomfortable.

Imitate the movements of other people, particularly those movements which seem to be least familiar or which you like least.

Feel how your body responds to them.

Let the movements slowly decrease, come to rest, breathe deeply.

Use music if you like for these exercises.

EXERCISES

FIVE EXERCISES DONE LYING DOWN

Lie on the floor on your back but raise your head, and if necessary chest, with wedge, cushion or blanket to avoid abdominal tension and heartburn.

1 Lift your legs and arms; move them in all directions (like a baby does).

2 With your legs in the air, circle your feet; move your toes; bend and stretch your legs.

3 On an inbreath, bend your knees, and put your feet on the floor.

On an outbreath, let your legs glide into a stretched position.

4 With your knees bent and feet a hand's width apart, glide your left hand down the left side of your body, or along the floor towards your foot.

On an inbreath, let the upper part of your body follow.

On an outbreath, let it relax back.

On the next inbreath, let the upper part of your body follow your hand down the right side on your body.

On the outbreath return.

5 Bend your knees, keep your feet close together with knees touching and breathe in.

Breathing out, put your bent legs on the floor on your right side.

Then, without moving your shoulders, while breathing in bring your legs back to the middle.

Now on the outbreath, place your bent legs to the left, then on the inbreath, bring them back.

Pause, then slowly roll over onto your side and using your hands and feet, get up in stages.

Exercises to loosen the pelvis

PAIR EXERCISE

TILTING THE PELVIS 1: STANDING ─────────

Stand up, with legs slightly bent and knees soft.

The partner puts his hands on the woman's tummy and bottom (above the pubic bone and at the height of the coccyx). The woman tilts her pelvis back and forward and finds a position for her pelvis, which feels comfortable and in which the baby rests in the pelvic frame, as if it were in a cradle. Neither abdomen nor spine are strained.

PAIR EXERCISE

TILTING THE PELVIS 2: LYING ─────────

Lie down with knees bent and feet on the floor. The partner puts his hands under the waist and the coccyx of the woman (the back of his hands to the floor).

His hands press alternately, she responds by pressing her body against the pressing hand, tilting her pelvis that way.

Now try the exercise with coordinated breathing. On the inbreath the woman presses her coccyx against her partner's hand; on the outbreath, she presses her waist against his hand.

This exercise is particularly suitable for participants who don't succeed in tilting their pelvis in a standing position.

EXERCISE

ROCKING THE PELVIS ─────────

This is particularly suitable for women who make only large or jerky movements.

Lie on the floor, become aware of how the whole of your back is touching the floor. Feel the floor beneath your legs, your arms, your head . . .

Now, pull your legs up, so that your knees are bent and the soles of your feet are flat on the floor. Your legs should be parallel, neither touching nor leaning outwards.

Now feel your legs. Start at the hip-joint.

Feel your thighs, go down to your knees . . . to your calves.

Feel your shinbones, your ankles, the soles of your feet.

Press slightly with your feet as if the floor beneath them was sand and could give way.

Feel how your feet are rooted in this ground beneath you.

Now become aware of your breathing.

Let the breath glide into your body, deep and relaxed.

With the next outbreath give a little push with your feet, and release with the inbreath.

Give pressure only with your feet, don't use your thighs or anything else.

Allow this pressure to come and go rhythmically with your breathing and feel the rhythm within your whole body.

Now slowly reduce the pressure with each outbreath and then stop.

Let your legs glide down again, so that they rest stretched and slightly apart.

EXERCISE

ROTATING THE PELVIS 1

This is a good exercise to massage yourself and relieve backache.

Lean against a wall with your feet about 8 in. away. Press your sacrum against the wall and make circles: to the right, upward, to the left, down.

Now, imagine a clock dial behind your pelvis: 12 o'clock is your waist, 3 o'clock your right side, 6 o'clock your coccyx and 9 o'clock your left side.

Make circles clockwise and anticlockwise. Repeat, so that on an inbreath your pelvis moves from 3 to 9 and on an outbreath, from 9 to 3.

EXERCISE

ROTATING THE PELVIS 2

Get down onto all fours.

Move your shoulders and pelvis to the right, and wag your body.

Move shoulders and pelvis to the left, wag your body.

Repeat this several times.

Rotate your pelvis: to the right with your back round; to the left with your back straight.

Repeat several times, taking care to only rotate the pelvis and not exaggerate the 'wagging' movements.

EXERCISE

LOOSENING THE GROIN

Lie on your back.

Draw the right leg up and lift the right half of your pelvis.

Turn your head to the left.

Now draw the left leg up, while the right leg remains bent, with both feet on the floot.

Lift the left side of the pelvis, and turn your head to the right.

Aim for flowing movements, accompanied by flowing breath. Find your own rhythm.

Come to rest.

Now lift the right half of the pelvis, while the head turns to the right.

Then lift the left half, the head turns left.

Let the breath flow with the movement.

Find your own rhythm.

Has anything changed?

EXERCISE

LOOSENING THE HIP JOINTS

Lie on your back.

Spread your relaxed arms and legs apart. Rotate them outwards with an inbreath, and rotate them inward with an outbreath.

Repeat this several times.

In the same relaxed spread-eagled position as above, shorten your stretched right leg (the right half of the pelvis is pulled up and breath) in.

Relax, let go, and breathe out.

Now, shorten your stretched left leg (pulling up the left half of the pelvis) and breathe in.

Relax, let go and breathe out.

Repeat several times.

EXERCISE ┌─ **STRETCHING** ───

(Valuable if you have got sciatic pain.) If these exercises cause you any discomfort – do not continue with them – always listen to the signals your body is giving you – all women are different. Different exercises suit different people.

Go down gently on all fours.

Make sure that your back is straight, change the distance between knees and arms if necessary.

With the inbreath stretch the right leg back.

Keep your head high, and your face pointing forward.

Keep the back stretched.

Now with the outbreath bring the leg in, and lower your head so that your face is pointing to your knee, and your back is rounded.

Repeat with left leg and then repeat, stretching both legs alternately.

EXERCISE ┌─ **BUTTERFLY POSITION** ──────────────────────────────────

Sit on the floor with the soles of your feet together, and your knees open.

Rock your knees towards the floor. Place your hands under your knees – or gently push them from above.

Try to touch the floor with your knees, alternating with the left and the right knee. Try not to lose your balance, and keep your back straight.

Rock your pelvis to and fro.

Feel the bones you sit on (the ischial tuberosities)

PAIR EXERCISE ┌─ **BUTTERFLY POSITION PAIR VARIANT** ──────────────────

Sit with your back well supported by cushions.

Place the soles of your feet together, and spread your knees apart.

Ask your partner to sit in front of you and to place his hands under your knees.

Let your legs vibrate.

Every now and then your partner should let go of your legs carefully, and let them drop a little bit further apart.

EXERCISE

SQUATTING

As with most of the other exercises, this one can be used to sensitize participants to the messages the body sends. Encourage participants to become aware of their different responses to pain, whether they are trying to avoid it, to fight it, to give in to it, or whether they are recognizing it as a valuable message from the body, not to go as far as that.

Squat down as far as possible with the soles of your feet on the floor. Try to gently move up and down while maintaining a squatting position.

The softening of the ligaments during pregnancy will help, so that soon everyone will be able to really squat down and to keep the legs closer together.

If it hurts stop.

If you are not used to squatting, start with support for your heels (folded blanket, books, a mat or high-heeled shoes). Squat, sway your pelvis alternating to the left and the right side.

EXERCISE

PELVIS SEE-SAW

An excellent and simple exercise to loosen the pelvis during birth and to keep the breath slow and in flow with the movements.

Standing, sitting or lying.

Suitable for all positions in birth.

Find your own breathing-rhythm. Rock the pelvis, following your breathing.

On the inbreath, arch your back; on the outbreath, make your back rounded.

EXERCISE ┌─ **LEG ROLLING** ─────────────────────

Duration: $1\frac{1}{2}$–2 min.

Goal of the exercise:

- to loosen the pelvis
- to allow pain and breathe with it
- to become more aware of the pelvis
- to simulate a contraction

Sit on the floor, your legs stretched and spread apart as far as possible.

Place your hands behind you on the floor for support.

Turn your feet outward, in a rolling movement that starts from the hip-joints.

Turn the feet inward, in a rolling movement, the hip-joint turns inward as well.

Now alternate: out, in; out, in. The emphasis is on the movement outward.

Carry on with the movement.

Let the movement become faster.

Take away the supporting hands, roll the legs: out, in . . .

Sit up straight.

Stretch your arms forward, to the sides, upward, and keep on rolling your legs.

Exercise the chest muscles – let your arms make circles, the legs stay with their movement: out, in . . .

Then support yourself with your hands again. Slow down the rolling movement of the legs, come to rest.

EXERCISE ┌─ **PELVIC 'SWING'** ──────────────────

When, during birth, the partner sees the woman stiffening her pelvis, he can step behind her as the contraction starts and help her to loosen her pelvis with rhythmic swinging.

Things which are tightly pressed together – the cork in the bottle-beck, the ring on the finger, the baby in the birth channel – detach most easily by rotation.

Often it is not enough for the woman to *know* that she should relax and keep her pelvis loose in labour.

As the contraction starts, there is a tendency to get tense, to tighten the pelvic muscles and to wait until 'it' is over.

Some women don't manage to let their pelvis move freely – neither during preparation nor during birth. It is of help, then, to suggest a rhythmic swing which the couple can learn together.

Both stand upright.

The partner stands close up behind the woman.

The woman's back touches the whole of the partner's front: his right leg being in touch and aligned with her right leg.

The partner leans slightly against the women so that she can lean against him too.

Both support the other, rather than the partner taking all the woman's weight.

The partner places his hands just above the woman's hip joints.

Pushing lightly he moves his pelvis against the woman, so that they move as one, as follows:
Inbreath: twice to the left, outbreath: twice to the right etc.

Each couple can find their own variation.

The pelvis can also be rocked forward and back or in a circling motion.

A different breathing rhythm can also be followed.
Inbreath – pelvis tilts back, outbreath – pelvic tilts forward. Or:
Inbreath: swing to the right; outbreath: swing to the left; whatever suits the couple.

Exercises for the pelvic floor

EXERCISES

FIVE EXERCISES FOR THE PELVIC FLOOR

Exercises 1–3 can be done in any position and should be practised as much as possible. Get into the habit of doing them whenever you are peeling the potatoes, at the bus stop . . . waiting for the kettle to boil, on the phone . . . whatever you would like use as a trigger.

Aims:

○ Improved blood flow to the muscles of the pelvic floor which then gain more elasticity. This, in turn, can help to prevent the likelihood of episiotomy.
○ Increased self-awareness (when am I tense?, when am I relaxed); valuable during second stage, and also during or after an internal check-up.

The third exercise usually doesn't work first time – to be able to do the exercise is one of its aims. The fourth exercise was developed according to the 'orgasm-reflex' of Dr. Wilhelm Reich. The fifth exercise is often experienced as quite intense. As homework the 3rd exercise is better suited because it can be done in any position and is therefore more likely to be practised.

Observe: What else do you tense up involuntarily? Abdomen, buttocks, thighs?

1 Any position standing, sitting or lying.

Relax your pelvic floor muscles by pretending to pass urine. Then tense the muscles gradually as though stopping the flow. Hold for a few seconds, then gradually relax the muscles to allow the 'flow' to continue.

Of course, this can be practised on the lavatory!

---

2 Tense the pelvic floor, a little bit more, even more, keep the tension, let go.

Breathe out and check if your pelvic floor is really relaxed again.

Take care, that despite the effort, the breathing is normal. Don't hold the breath!

---

3 Imagine your pelvic floor as a lift.

Normal relaxation of the pelvic floor is the ground floor. Now go to the first floor, the second, the third and finally the fourth floor.

On every floor increase the tension a little and hold it for a moment.

Now go down again: to the third floor, the second floor, the first floor and lastly back to the ground floor.

As you descend to each floor release the tension a little.

Try to reach the basement.

Your vulva will be protruding slightly.

Place your hand over your pelvic floor to check for the bulging.

---

4 This exercise, reminiscent perhaps of the sexual act, offers the experience of how much we are prepared to open up and to give in to the birth process.

Lie on the floor, feet on the ground, knees bent and slightly apart.

Let your breath flow slowly and deeply.

Add a new movement after every 4–5 breaths so that in the end five different motions are done simultaneously – as if the body is rolled over by waves, to and fro . . . as follows:

1 Inbreath:	1 Outbreath:
2 Tense the pelvic floor	2 Relax pelvic floor
3 Arch your back	3 Press round of back into floor
4 Bring the knees together	4 Let your knees sink apart
5 Bring the chin to the chest	5 Bend your head back

closing   opening

5 Duration: 3–5 min.

On all fours with rounded back.

Breathe deep into your tummy, try to reach the pelvic floor with your breath.

Tense the muscles around the urethra (urinal opening) as if you would interrupt the flow of urine, let go.

Now tense and relax the muscles around your anus.

Continue to breathe in a relaxed way.

Tense and release the muscles around your vagina, without interrupting your flow of breath.

Now tense all the muscles of the pelvic floor.

Draw them inside and hold.

Draw them higher and higher and higher.

Breathe in a very relaxed way into your abdomen and down to the pelvic floor. Feel the warmth of the blood circulating round the pelvic area and pelvic floor.

Draw your muscles in even higher.

Hold the tension.

Continue to breathe in a very relaxed way.

Then, gently, let go.

This second part of the exercise is suitable as a stress-exercise.

Again contract all the muscles of the pelvic floor.

Breathe relaxedly, in and out.

Now, contract the muscles even more, draw them inside; continue to breathe relaxedly, but hold the tension.

Contract the muscles even more.

Continue to breathe in a very relaxed way.

Then, gently, let go.

Become very soft and relaxed.

Move your pelvis.

Become aware of the warmth and relaxation of the pelvic floor.

19 Touch relaxation and massage

REFLECTIONS It is fashionable to offer touch relaxation and massage in antenatal courses. In some course-plans they occupy a relatively large amount of time, even though quite a lot of women don't want to be touched at all while giving birth. Others enjoy it in antenatal classes, as they receive an amount of attention and tenderness through it that they would miss out on otherwise.

As facilitators we have to be clear what we want to achieve with touch relaxation and massage in the course. First, we should ask ourselves:
   – what roles do touch relaxation and massage play in the preparation for birth?
   – what contribution can they make to labour and birth?
   – how important are they in our life with our partners?
   – how important are they in our courses?

Then, we should consider whether touch, relaxation and massage is:
   – a technique which could be helpful during birth?
   – a way of making the partners more sensitive to each other (indirect preparation)?
   – a positive experience for the women?

It is very important that giving and receiving are evenly distributed. The men should get as much attention as the women, so that they don't feel that they are required to give only. Ina May Gaskins in *Spiritual Midwifery* suggests that the women are asked to massage their partners during the birth, the idea being that not only receiving but also giving loosens tension. For most exercises, it is a good idea to let the women practise on the men first. Then they can give the TR and massage the way they would like to receive it. Often the women are more sensitive than the men. If women massage first, a lot of mistakes can be avoided which could happen, if the men began first, although the reverse can also be true.

When presenting the exercises, talk about giving and receiving. Good TR or massage depends not only on the way the partner gives it, but also on how the recipient receives it:
– can I allow myself to be touched?
– can I accept that somebody is giving me something, doing me good?

Do I close myself, out of an old – and may be no longer valid – experience, that what I get isn't the right thing anyway?
– am I somebody, nobody can serve properly?

Such reflections are more important than learning a massage technique. Quite often during birth the energy doesn't flow, it gets stuck somehow, and the cervix stops opening because the woman closes herself to the caresses of her partner, or because the man doesn't respond to her attention and caresses.

Touch relaxation exercises

EXERCISE

PREPARATION

The partner lies or leans back comfortably so that the woman has access to him from all round.

The partner breathes in a relaxed way and anticipates being touched.

The woman becomes calm. She focuses on her own breathing. She sits relaxed.

The woman observes where her partner is tense.

She gently ascertains, where it feels right to touch her partner.

She places a hand with a conscious approach, carefully reaching into the 'aura' of her partner, feeling the 'cushion of air' around.

The woman touches her partner lightly, on her outbreath.

She then lets her hand become heavier.

The partner surrenders to the touch: he takes in the hand; he offers no resistance.

He imagines his breath flowing to the place where the woman's hand touches.

Body positions and the areas maximally receptive to touch relaxation.

Lying on side	Shoulders, back, buttocks, outside of the thighs, feet.
Sitting	Temples, forehead, jaws, shoulders, belly, pubic area.

| All-fours | Shoulders, back, arms, outside of the thighs, buttocks. |
| Lying on back | Pelvic floor (see page 148). |

EXERCISES

FOUR VARIATIONS OF TOUCH RELAXATION

Exercises 1 and 2, ideally, should be practised as much as possible and whenever necessary in everyday life. They should be done mutually so that they become almost a reflex to release tense shoulders, frowning etc.

Exercises 3 and 4 are particularly suitable during labour, especially if the woman starts to lose her breathing rhythm. If she starts to breath in a hectic way, she can be led back to her natural rhythm without words, just by stroking. This demands considerable sensitivity of the partner as he needs to find out when it is right for the woman to slow down her breathing or when to speed it up.

1 The partner places his hand on the woman, and lets it sink in.

The woman imagines her breath to reach the place where her partner's hand is, and becomes aware of this place.

The partner lifts his hand carefully and softly.

The woman imagines the touched place to melt as the hand becomes lighter.

She lets go of tension.

Images: the softness of a rising yeast dough.
The melting of a ripe camembert.

2 The partner places his hand on the woman, giving light pressure.

The woman relaxes into the pressure.

The partner leaves his hand where it is until he feels the tension is melting, then he strokes the tension out, taking it away.

To avoid blockages he strokes the whole arm and hand: the whole leg and foot; the whole trunk.

The woman surrenders and allows her tension to be taken away.

3 The partner places his hand on the woman.

To begin with his touch is light; he observes her breathing.

Then, with her inbreath his touch becomes softly pressured.

With her outbreath, his touch lightens again. His hand remains in contact with her body all the time.

4 The partner breathes slowly and deeply.

With the outbreath the woman applies long langorous strokes down the partner's back; down the arm, down the leg; all the while emphasizing the outbreath, the relaxation, the letting go.

Repeat each exercise with changed roles.

EXERCISE
Touch relaxation

WHEN THE CHILD IS IN BREECH POSITION

The partner kneels on the floor, a cushion between the heels and the buttocks.

The woman lies on her back in front of him.

She comes closer with her buttocks and places the hollows of her knees on his shoulders.

Both come even closer together.

He on his knees, she wriggling with her shoulders, until her pelvis rests on his thighs.

They stay in this position for 10 minutes.

Both think of the child.

Both wish the child to turn.

The partner touches, strokes, relaxes the belly of the woman, coaxing the child.

She breathes deeply and in a relaxed way, widening the abdominal cavity. They can stay in this position for as long as they are both comfortable. When they want to end the exercise, the partner wriggles his knees out from under her buttocks and she rolls over to her side getting up slowly via the all-fours position in order not to strain her abdominal muscles.

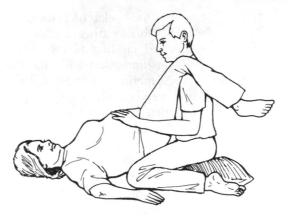

Massage

Massage which might be helpful during birth

Most women don't want a full massage during birth (kneading treatment of the buttocks, thighs or shoulders), but some do. For most, touch relaxation works best as a nonverbal way of releasing tense parts of the body, and is the 'utmost' external sensation that can be tolerated because so much is happening inside. Very light stroking of the belly is sometimes wanted and experienced as comfortable.

However, circling movements can stimulate contractions (see Fig. a). If contractions are very strong, the movements/circles should be interrupted to achieve relaxation. (see Figs b and c)

The stroking movements shown in figures b and c can also include caressing of the breasts and nipples and/or clitoris. The caressing movements will not only enhance the stimulation of the clitoris, lead to wellbeing but will stimulate the release of more oxytocin and stronger contractions.

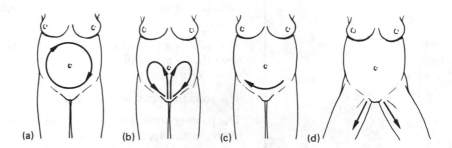

(a)   (b)   (c)   (d)

Back massage

Many women experience contractions as backache, particularly when the baby is presenting posteriorly. With every contraction the head of the child is pressed against the spine. This is known as 'backache labour'.

As the backache is increased if the woman lies on her back or leans back whilst sitting, a change of position often brings relief. Leaning forward, circling movements of the pelvis, going down on all-fours are all positions that will take the pressure off the spine.

Sometimes it feels as if the pressure of the baby's head will burst the pelvis. When this happens, it is helpful if counterpressure is applied. This necessitates the cooperation of the partner – sometimes for hours!

The massaging partner should sit or stand comfortably, and use his body weight to apply counterpressure, so that he is not straining his arm muscles. It is important to ask where counterpressure is wanted, as the pressure of the baby's head gradually shifts down to the coccyx. The pressure can be applied with the palm of one hand (the other hand supports), or with the fist or the knuckles – whatever feels better for both partners. Press with slow circling movements: the muscles should be moved on the bones; don't rub the skin. That could cause irritation of the skin – particularly if it is done for hours. Sometimes the partner kneels behind the labouring woman applying counterpressure in the right place with his hands – or alternatively they could sit back to back with one another his back providing the counterpressure.

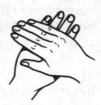

EXERCISE

MASSAGE TO RELAX THE PELVIC FLOOR

A very simple response can be learned.

The woman lies on her back or takes a half-sitting position (as for perhaps, second stage or an internal check-up), allowing the legs to fall open.

The partner strokes the inside of the thighs from the knees towards the pelvic floor. He uses light strokes or strong pressure, whatever is wanted.

The woman tenses her pelvic floor.

The partner strokes from the pelvis down to the knees, again, lightly or firmly, whatever is wanted.

The woman relaxes her pelvic floor.

After a couple of times the relaxation response occurs almost automatically. Then the upward strokes and the deliberate contraction can be left out. The partner can help the woman to relax at any time when she feels that she is tensing her pelvic floor.

EXERCISE

> ### FOOT MASSAGE
>
> TO AVOID AND HELP TO PREVENT VARICOSE VEINS AND ŒDEMA
>
> The partner sits comfortably on a stool, chair or the edge of a bed.
>
> The woman lies in front of him on the floor. If necessary the upper part of her body is supported by a cushion. Her feet are lying in the partner's lap.
>
> The partner massages the soles of the woman's feet, every toe, the ankles, the lower calves, with circling fingers. Strong pressure on the feet is often experienced as very pleasurable.

EXERCISE

> ### LEG MASSAGE
>
> The partner sits on the floor or leans against a wall, supported by a cushion.
>
> The woman lies on the floor; if necessary, her upper body is supported by a cushion.
>
> She places her feet on the partner's shoulders.
>
> The partner strokes the woman's legs from the feet to the buttocks. First, one whole leg with both hands; then both legs, with the hands on the outside of the legs (don't work on individual varicosities).
>
> The strokes should be firm to begin with; then become lighter.

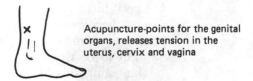

Acupuncture-points for the genital organs, releases tension in the uterus, cervix and vagina

As homework, the couples can try the different massage strokes or touch relaxations experimenting with oil and lotion, or talk to see what suits them best.

20 Positions in childbirth

REFLECTIONS **1** How important is it for you that women should use certain positions during labour and for giving birth?
– what are your experiences?
– which positions did you use when you gave birth?

2 Some midwives, doctors and antenatal teachers have very fixed ideas about labouring and delivery positions. Often this is because they have learned about certain positions during their training and never questioned them or experienced the effectiveness of alternative positions. Do you have such fixed ideas?

3 Have you noticed that even in the 'natural birth scene' one frequently finds a group pressure on labouring women to use certain positions? Although these positions might have their advantages, as long as they just become a new norm, they are no better than the traditional ones.

4 Every birth is different: a position that could be effective for one woman becomes a hindrance for another. It is most important that pregnant women and couples are not taught certain positions, thought to be right for certain stages in labour.

The aim should be for women and couples to acquire body self-awareness, so that they can feel for themselves which position is right for them at any given time.

If a woman is taught to be upright during second stage (possibly even in a specific position), yet the midwife tells her to lie down in such and such a position, the two opinions clash, and the woman is left to choose between two conflicting authorities at a time when her energies are better used in actively going with her body in the labouring process.

○ She might choose to follow the authority of a book or her antenatal teacher and feel fine or

○ She might choose to follow the authority of a book or her antenatal teacher, ignoring her own body's current needs and impede her labour process by working against her body.

If the woman developed self-awareness during her pregnancy, she is likely to know which position her body needs to be in.

But there are subtle differences in listening to ourselves. We can listen to our own stubbornness:

Flexibility is more important than any rule

Jenny was fixed on the idea that she wanted to give birth in a squatting position. She was impressed by a film she saw. It made sense to her on a mental level. She had trained her body to be able to squat comfortably. Second stage came and she squatted. Nothing happened. There was no progress. Everything seemed transfixed. Her motives. Her decision. Her position. Her baby. As soon as she allowed herself to lie down, the baby was quickly born.

We can listen to our own weakness:

Rosemary was lying exhausted on the bed in second stage. Nothing progressed. The baby's head did not descend. Contractions weakened. She was encouraged to get up just for a few contractions. She declined: 'Oh no, I couldn't. Let me lie, I'm much too exhausted'. But really, she had to find her own strength again. One part of her had given up. Supported on both sides, she was got out of bed and encouraged to move her pelvis around. The contractions picked up in strength, and the baby's head soon became visible. After a few contractions the process had been established and she was helped back onto the bed again to give birth.

We can listen to our body despite 'better' knowledge:

When it came to my own first labour I found myself lying face down on my bed. Contractions had just overwhelmed me, so it seemed. I had never heard of anybody lying face down in labour and certainly 'knew' about the advantages of an upright position. When the midwife came and examined me it soon became clear why my body wanted to lie that way. My baby had disengaged himself again and was now in posterior presentation. Lying on my tummy encouraged his little back to move sideways. Which he did within a few hours.
Being upright just would not have helped us at all, as his head would have been pressed against my pelvic frame, unable to move any further down.

Kate stamped up and down the hall in transition. The midwives all 'knew' it might be easier for her to lie on her side or to keep her bottom higher than her chest to relieve the pressure of the baby's head. Yet she knew that she had to get rid of excess energy before she could settle down to give birth.

On one of the first 'natural labours' I experienced, the woman was lying in bed on her back, just relaxing, breathing. I was aghast she was too laid back for my ideals, and what about the supine hypotensive syndrome? But she seemed so comfortable and labour was progressing well, so she was left to lie. This was supposed to be that special natural birth. In fact this woman had flown over from America to give birth. She knew all about birth positions, had especially chosen a 'progressive' midwife. Yet obviously she was in touch with her body too. The whole labour and birth only lasted three hours, and she was a 35-year-old primigravida! I am still ashamed that I had almost encouraged her to get up and move about. She knew what was right for her. She trusted her body.

A vast range of labouring positions can be suggested and explored in the antenatal class, and participants encouraged to try out new variations at home. Here are some guidelines for women and couples to find their own positions, those with which they feel comfortable and which they might or might not use during labour. Any of the listed additional advantages are overruled by the woman's sense of well-being. The emphasis is always on being open and flexible. Any position in which the woman is comfortable and labour progresses is right. It is more important that the woman feels that she can relax, let go and give in to the birth process, than it is for her to be in a physically optimal position.

Guidelines for positions in labour

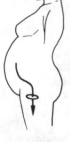

First stage   The position should be such that

- Woman feels comfortable
- Back is rounded forward (with an arched back the baby has to combat one more curve)

wrong

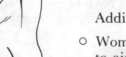

right

Additionally:

- Woman can move her pelvis freely (to keep the pelvis loose and to aid the baby's descent)
- Weight of the baby's head or buttocks presses onto the cervix to stimulate its opening (physically and hormonally)
- Weight of the baby does *not* press onto the back (could lead to back ache and supine hypotensive syndrome)

Transition The position should be
- as above, except
- Baby's head need not press onto the cervix anymore.

Additionally,

- Cervix (in the pelvis) kept temporarily higher than the baby (in the abdomen) to avoid unnecessary pressure and pushing urge.

Second stage

The position should be such that

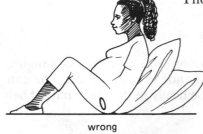

wrong

- Woman does *not* sit on her coccyx (as this narrows the birth passage)
- Woman does not arch her back (see first stage position)

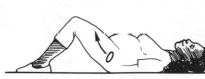

right

- Woman does not sit in a deep squat (the birth passage is narrower then, than in any other position and the pelvis isn't as flexible).

Additionally,

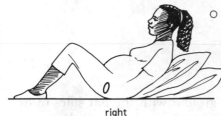

unfavourable

- Woman is not lying flat (otherwise the baby has to move upwards)
- Weight of the baby pushes downwards using gravity

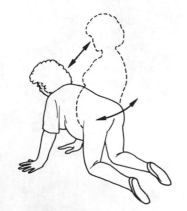

- Pelvis can be moved freely (circling of the pelvis aids the internal rotation and descent of the baby)

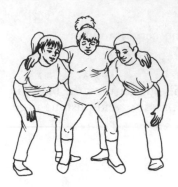

○ Woman can be supported and held by one or two people in a standing or semi-squatting position

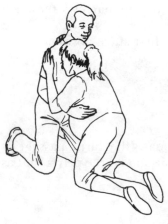

○ Woman while standing, kneeling or semi-squatting is hanging onto a partner or a frame with hands or arms so that she can allow herself to really open and be heavy in the lower part of her body.

○ Woman stands firmly on the ground with the flat soles of her feet to feel her own stability, strength and groundedness.

PART 3 The Psychological Aspects of Pregnancy and Childbirth

---

21 Psychological and emotional aspects of pregnancy and childbirth

To conceive, grow and give birth to a child are both incredibly profound and emotive experiences. What's more, they touch everything in our lives. There are:

○ Body changes
Within weeks of conception, breasts will be increasing in size and we may notice a thickening waistline. Gradually the growing roundness calls for a change in dressing and becomes obvious to outsiders. Our centre of gravity shifts and with it posture. There are too the symptoms of pregnancy: fatigue, nausea, frequency etc.
During labour the body takes over in overpowering sensation.

○ Lifestyle changes
There is a need to slow down: to appraise values and priorities. Work is tailored to suit our capacity.
Fatigue limits social life, and interests shift as resting instinct develops.
Prospect of child may cause tremendous drive and motivation to 'get things (often long put-off) done'.

○ Relationship changes
partner:
Couple to develop into family.
There may be a change in sexual needs and responses.
Prospect of financial dependency may pressure and/or motivate partner.
Expectations and tastes demand appraisal and adaptation.

Friends:
Some became more important than others as our needs change

Parents:
There might be a shift of attention away from us towards the baby. We might suddenly be able to set boundaries, protect our baby more than we were able to protect ourselves from their interference. Or we might become less critical of their parenting and more appreciative of what they have done for us.

Other children:
Reappraise our treatment of them. We might give them more freedom than before just because we haven't got the time, we might find ourselves reacting more strictly than before because we are strained. We might neglect them or pamper them because of their loss of 'status' (the only one, the youngest one, the only boy – girl etc.).

○ Emotional changes.
Fear	what is to come, the unknown, loneliness, pain, inadequacy, handicap, lack of love etc.
Anger	towards childbirth professionals, partner, colleagues, parents, society at large
Envy	friends without children, those with money, other pregnant women, mothers who seem to have a better lot.
Anxiety:	about the future; one's looks, health, money, lifestyle matters etc.

Sadness about the loss of independence, freedom etc.

In addition to the emotional corollaries of the above, there may be overwhelming feelings as we realize the enormity of what has happened (conception) and all that is to come. Many, ostensibly paradoxical feelings may be jostling side by side for supremacy. There may be euphoria mixed in doubt and ambivalence; anger and vulnerability. Strength and fear.

And however well we are coping and adapting, however happy we are about all the changes, however strongly we wanted them to happen there is always loss involved. Saying goodbye to a phase of our life that was without children, taking leave of the 'me' that was 'just' wife, lover, daughter etc. and not yet mother. Even saying goodbye to the pregnancy if the roundness of it all was pleasurable. In many respects, pregnancy and childbirth are a rite of passsage carrying us from the realm of girlhood to the wider, more profound world of womanhood. The sense of loss may feel very real, and there may even be a need to grieve for what now has to be left behind.

Our role as antenatal teachers

On the one hand   – feelings might be better untouched as they could erupt!

> — we are not qualified therapists
> — even if we were, pregnant couples don't come to us for therapy (it is not our contract)

and yet
> — the emotional aspects are inseparable from body and mind
> — we cannot prepare for birth purely mentally or physically
> — sound emotions are the basis for a good birth experience.
> — pregnant couples usually have nowhere else to go to with their fears and worries

So what is our role?

Not to analyse!
Not to operate!
Not to theorize!
We are *not* responsible for their emotions
We do not need to change their feelings

> turning fear into confidence
> envy into admiration
> hate into compassion

They do not need to change their feelings
Can we accept that it is OK to feel frightened?!
> angry?!
> envious?!

How do we feel ourselves as childbirth professionals?

(not to mention all the feelings of our private realm)
We might feel joy and satisfaction (birth experience, contact with people etc).
We might feel anger, boredom and frustration (the unfavourable hospital system, the repetition of the theme).
We might feel fear (of disappointment, complications, failure).
We might feel envy (of pregnancy, birthing and breastfeeding, of better work situations elsewhere).
We have needs in our work too (to be loved, to be needed, to prove ourselves).

REFLECTIONS 1 What are your basic feelings and beliefs as a childbirth professional? What subconscious messages do you convey? For example, that:
> — giving birth is very complicated; to achieve natural birth, takes a lot of preparation?

– giving birth is easy: everybody can have a natural birth; those who can't must be neurotic?
– 'You can try, but it probaby won't work anyway with our present hospital situation?'
– 'You must try, you must prove it is possible, otherwise I have failed as an antenatal teacher, midwife etc.?'

2 Can you be honest about your own emotions? (Self-awareness)
Can you accept that you have negative emotions too? (Self-acceptance)
Can you allow yourself to ask for what you need? (Self-assertiveness)

3 Focus on what you are feeling right now. Use the following exercise. First, settle comfortably, breathe out, relax as much as your body allows you to.

Always be aware and stay in touch with your own feelings when working with other people's feelings

Let yourself know which parts of your body feel uncomfortable, still tense, tight or cold.
Try shifting around a bit and breathing out, sighing, a couple of times.
Let your body know that you are receiving and acknowledging its signals.

Now look at all the parts of your body that feel good: warm, soft, relaxed, and comfortable.
Wriggle about a bit if you like, or just stay with that well-being for a while.
Enjoy your breathing and your relaxed position.

Now, let yourself feel what has been going on inside you, these last few days; and today, and right now.
What feelings are in the foreground? What feelings are in the background?
Scan the whole range of your feelings and the whole spectrum of emotions that is part of you.
Sort them through as if you are packing a suitcase.
Put aside all those feelings that don't belong to your professional self and that you don't want to deal with right now.
Breathe out and let go with each outbreath.
Stay aware of all the feelings that influence your work as a childbirth professional.
Stretch, yawn, sigh. Make a few notes perhaps.

If we are honest and open with our own feelings we can then encourage group participants to acknowledge their own feelings. Equally, if we allow ourselves to have negative feelings and to accept their validity, we can allow and accept that group participants also have negative feelings. In this way we take responsibility for ourselves and also do not become distracted with ideals and unrealistic expectations. We can inspire and encourage participants to start taking care of their own needs.

Our own messages and responses are the key. We are influential — and that brings responsibility, i.e. a mother feels guilty because she finds her baby ugly, having been told every mother thinks her own child the most beautiful. It might be a result of her contact with us whether or not a woman sees herself as a good enough mother.

It is important to talk about the validity of negative emotions in antenatal classes and to be allowed to express them. (Studies of postnatal depression show that the more fear and anxiety expressed before birth, the less postnatal depression took place.) Anger helps us work through grieving and loss (be it just the loss of our independence) and motivates us to make any changes. Feeling sad helps us to get in contact with our needs and desires. Fear and anxiety prepare us to deal with stressful situations. On a hormonal level, production of fight-or-flight adrenalin makes us physically stronger to face our adversary.

Emotional expression in antenatal classes

How *we* react to feelings that are expressed in antenatal visits or classes is equally important. Whether *we* demean, belittle or encourage them. We should also be aware how the couple respond to one another. How does the partner react if his/her other half expresses pain, fear, anger etc?

EXAMPLE

Husband expresses fear about possible complications at home delivery:
   – is the wife 'infected' by his fear?
   – because he does all the worrying for her does she feel even more secure?
   – does she keep her feelings in check?

Wife expresses fear about possible complications at home delivery:
   – does he try to blackmail her (but you always wanted . . .) pushes her to go through with it?
   – does he talk her out of it, belittles her fear?
   – does he take the decision not to have a home delivery instead of talking through her fears with her?

The above examples are the usual response patterns. (Of course it is possible for the man too to respond in a 'self-directed' way and for the woman to respond in an 'other-directed' way.)

If we observe any of these responses we can tactfully point out what we perceive, without judgement. We can also demonstrate that it is possible to respond differently: to listen to and accept the emotions without being affected by them, and without needing to attack or belittle them. We can encourage partners to reformulate their response into an 'I' statement, which also encourage the person to 'own' and take responsibility for his/her feelings. For example:

'I get very confused when I hear your fears, because I am not so sure myself whether it is the right thing, let's talk about all the pros and cons again.'

or

'I am very confident that home birth is the right choice. What has happened that triggered those fears in you, let's talk about it.'

May be they could try a couple of reformulation versions until it feels right to them.

Until he or she feels it expresses honestly where they are at, and it contains no more accusation or patronizing.

Possibly it just needs the suggestion from our part for the couple to explore the reformulation with each other.

Maybe it needs our help, in that we express our observations when it feels not quite clear to us. So we give an example how to clarify communication and we convey that there is nothing wrong or dangerous about expressing emotions.

What is important though, is that all this doesn't develop into a full-blown therapeutic session with one particular couple within the class.

Practising to say 'I' instead of 'you'

It only takes a few minutes to ask somebody in class to reformulate a sentence they have just said into an 'I' statement. It is a learning experience for the whole class. We all have to learn to be more honest and open with ourselves.

Another common response which can be reformulated, usually concerns what other people do to us.

For example:
'He hurts me.'
'He never listens to me.'
'You are threatening me.'
'She leaves all the talking to me.'

Instead of feeling we are the victims, we can turn our response round and acknowledge *our* role in the situation.

'I let him hurt me.'
'I cannot get my message across.'
'I feel threatened by you.'
'I do all the talking for her' etc.

Again, this is about taking responsibilities for our feelings.

To respond from ourselves, as class leaders, and to encourage communication in the class and within the couple, does not need any preparation or structure, it only requires for us to be in touch with ourselves.

22 Group leadership and group dynamics

How much group discussion and process you want to encourage or structure, will depend on your aims for your antenatal classes. It is not just a question of how much you know about group leadership and group dynamics, or what type of work suits your personality; it is more a question of What is your aim? What do you want to achieve in your work?

Once you have clarified your aims, the next step is to be able to *declare* them. People should know what to expect when they book for your classes. The third step is to establish a clear contract of 'service' with the participants on the first evening. Although antenatal classes have a therapeutic benefit, they are not a therapy group; if you are interested in the latter then call it a therapy group and establish a different contract with the participants.

Ask yourself:
– how capable and interested am I in establishing contact with pregnant mums and dads?
– what is my aim for the group and for the individual participant?
– can I formulate my aims clearly, so that participants understand what I mean?
– with which methods of group leadership and group dynamics do I feel at ease/ill at ease?

Introduce only those methods of group dynamics with which you feel easy; introduce only issues that you have worked through yourself, introduce only those exercises that you have tried out yourself and that you enjoy doing and, introduce them only when necessary.

Exercise can help you to structure the group and the theme. Be aware, when a group runs well and doesn't need any crutches.

The advantages of using group dynamic methods:

○ An issue can be dealt with in a much shorter time (15 minutes of structured exercise instead of 1 hour group discussion).
○ Everybody will contribute something (not only two or three as often happens in group discussions).
○ Participants experience it as more effective, as the structure helps to stay with the issue (instead of branching out into other themes as is often the case in group discussion).

It is important not to structure the group continuously, with one exercise after the other, without trust that the group can develop on its own.

The more freely you work the more time you need so that the participants can find their own way in the group discussions. Your role is then to ensure that all the participants have the opportunity to say what they want to say and that each theme or issue comes to a conclusion, with you giving a brief summary of the group discussion. Remember: to conclude a group discussion satisfactorily does not necessarily mean that everybody agrees. You can summarize by listing the different points of view and thus encourage continuing discussion outside the class. It is a pity when a couple returns home from an antenatal class satiated with nothing left to be said.

Exercises are like crutches – you have to know when to use them

The exercises on the following pages do not *have* to be part of an antenatal class. They are crutches. Some group constellations need more, other need less; some group leaders need more, others need less. And using crutches can be fun for all as long as you know that you don't really need them.

When using any of the exercises, do not aim to unearth any unconscious material nor to offer a solution for all problems. All the exercises have one thing in common, and it is always good to mention this when introducing them:

We can practise listening! Not only listening to our partners, or to other points of view, but also listening to ourselves!
  – what do I say with my words?
  – which thoughts find expression? (Which do not)?
  – what do I really mean?

To really listen to oneself, to grant importance to what one says, enables us to listen to others and to grant their expressions importance too.

Exercises for group participation

Introductions

The first round of introductions will be a stressful situation; even for those of us who are used to introducing ourselves and speaking in a group, this first introduction of ourselves is like a small birth. We

Introducing ourselves is a bit like giving birth

know it will be our turn sooner or later. The tension and apprehension increases the longer we have to wait for our turn. Or we might be relieved that we are not the next one yet. We can't really concentrate anymore on what the people before us say. And then suddenly it is our turn. There is enormous energy in us, increased heartbeat and blood pressure, flushed face, hardly any breath left – sometimes more, sometimes less. We probably have certain ideas about what we want to say, and hear ourselves saying them — finding it to our liking or feeling it to be quite awful — or we hear ourselves saying something completely different and feel pleased or embarrassed about that. Or we can't remember any of our plans for an introduction, stutter, 'abort', need 'forceps' in form of questions. Similarly, our partner might say something that surprises us or disappoints us. Afterwards we might judge ourselves and our partner's introduction differently again. It might cease to matter, or we hang on to our resentment. Are we the type of person who is satisfied in retrospect whatever happens? Are we critical and judgemental and never satisfied? Maybe we didn't have any plan of how to introduce ourselves and regret that now, or are pleased about that.

All these patterns of attitude and behaviour have their parallel when it comes to birth. We can use the first round of introduction as a stress situation and encourage, after the introduction round, the participants to reflect how they dealt with it. Maybe they will discover about themselves, that they were happy with the way they dealt with it. Maybe they want to explore different behaviour patterns next time round and there will be many occasions in the course of the classes. We can change if we want to! And discovering that we show one pattern in one situation, though it might teach us something about ourselves, does not mean we will, or have to, display the same pattern next time.

EXERCISE

SUGGESTIONS FOR THE INTRODUCTION ROUND ___

Choose whichever method suits your style and your group's needs.

INTRODUCING YOUR NAME (TWO VARIATIONS)

Sit in a circle

- ○ Everyone in turn (clockwise) talk a bit about your name — who gave it to you, why, what you know about it, whether you like it, what you would rather be called. (This also leads to thoughts of names for the child.)

- ○ Everybody in turn make a small gesture or movement — that is typical for you — sitting or standing up (possible stepping forward) while saying your name.

This avoids having to use many words, encourages body language, helps the other participants to remember the name.

REMEMBERING PARTICIPANTS' NAMES

○ After everyone has introduced him- or herself, one person starts: 'I am Gerlinde, you are Hilary; and the others follow: 'I am Hilary, you are Bridget; 'I am Bridget, you are . . .' and so on.

Another possibility is to, for a few who want, try to name everyone in the group!

○ In the second session, remind each other of your names and bring in an element of singing making sounds.
Everyone in turn sing his or her own name.
The whole group repeat it in a chorus.
With the next outbreath everybody sing his/her own variation of that name — higher, lower or with different intonation.

The ensuing disharmony is an important learning experience: Can I stick to my own sound even if it does not seem to fit?

INTRODUCTION WITHOUT INTERACTION (THREE VARIATIONS)

○ Everybody can say what they want. Participants will tend to copy the points the antenatal teacher or first person in the circle has covered, so for it to be effective, it needs a very aware and self-confident group.

○ Introduce yourselves — by name, occupation, age, children, expected date of delivery, pregnancy so far, home or hospital confinement, which hospital etc. . . . whatever you think the group wants to know about each other [Starting with the antenatal teacher].

○ One by one, tell the group something about yourself that has nothing to do with pregnancy or birth [This can be quite a challenge for most groups, but speeds up the group process — if that is what you want].

INTRODUCTION WITH INTERACTION (THREE VARIATIONS)

○ *A Cocktail Party*

Everyone [antenatal teacher included] get up and walk freely about, saying hello to everyone else and introducing your name and something about yourself.

○ *Variation*

Everybody introduce yourself to everyone else saying your name and asking one — any — question to the other person.

○ *Interview*

Everybody turn to your neighbour (not your own partner) and interview this person for 2–5 minutes.

Afterwards, everybody introduce your neighbour to the group with what you can remember from the 'interview'.

[Most people find it easier to introduce somebody else, not themselves, but it can be confusing to remember which bit of information belongs to whom, also some participants like to be responsible for their own introduction.]

REFLECTIVE QUESTIONING IN THE CIRCLE

○ Survey the other participants in the group, and ask yourself: What would I like to know from so-and-so? With whom would I like contact? Who am I not so interested in? Who do I dare ask something of? What would I like to know that I don't dare to ask? Which questions do I find easy to ask?

Then everybody reflect quietly on these questions. There is no discussion. After a short while, everybody is then able to ask somebody else what he or she wants to, although she doesn't have to. Neither do those asked a question, need to answer that particular one. They can let it be known what they would like to tell about themselves, and so respond to the question with: 'I would much rather tell you . . .'.

REFLECTIVE REPORTING IN THE CIRCLE

○ Survey the other participants, and ask yourself: What would I like to tell them about myself? What do I want them to know? Who in the group hinders me from telling specific things? What would I like to tell so-and-so, but not the others?

Everybody reflect quietly without *needing* to act — although there is the chance afterwards to say what you *want* to say.

THEME-SPECIFIC QUESTIONING (TWO VARIATIONS)

○ Begins by asking a specific question to one person. (This is after the introduction of names and/or the introduction without interaction.) For example:
  'Ann, what difficulties have you experienced in your pregnancy so far?' or:
  'Ann, how do you feel when you think about the hospital/midwife of your choice?'
  Ann then answers and asks the same question to somebody else in the group whose name she remembers.

○ In the second session this 'questioning' can be played slightly differently: everybody can ask anyone else in the group any one question. Each person who answered the

question addressed to him or her then asks someone else
another question.

George did you decide which clinic you will be going to?
(Answer) Janet, what happened at your last antenatal
check up?
(Answer) John did you go along to the ultrasound scan?
etc.

NO INTRODUCTION ROUND

This is possible too. You may believe that personal information
and exchange is not necessary for your type of course syllabus or
that you don't have to structure anything as personal interaction
happens by itself. In which case your course syllabus will be
loosely planned with enough breaks for interpersonal exchange
and process to take place spontaneously without any structure.

Further suggestions for the first session

EXERCISE

ROOM AWARENESS

Everyone stand in a circle and take off your shoes.

Find a comfortable standing position. Loosen yourself up a bit,
stretch, move your body gently, slowly begin to walk around the
room, observing the room as you walk about:
  – what can you see?
  – what do you like to look at in this room?
  – what do you dislike about it?
  – which features in this room are pleasant?
  – can you find a point where your eyes can rest?

  how does floor feel — soft? hard? cold? warm?
    – are there differences?
    – how do *you* feel?
    – what is different when you close your eyes?
    – what can you sense with your skin?
    – what can you hear?
    – what can you smell?
    – how do you feel about the things you sense, hear and
      smell?

Now open your eyes again and look for a place in the room
where you would like to sit. Arrange this particular place
for yourself comfortably with cushions, mat and blanket.

Reflection

How was this exercise for you? What effect has a new
room/environment on you? How strongly are you influenced
by new settings? Consider your responses in relation to the
labour ward birthing room.

EXERCISE ┌─ **DAY AWARENESS** ──────────────────

Possible at the beginning of each session.

Find a comfortable position on your chair or cushion.

Close your eyes if you want too.

Breathe in and out deeply and audibly.*

Let go of any accumulated tension with an audible outbreath.

Breathe in and out audibly, sighing between breaths. Let the tension melt away.

Slowly your body will feel softer and you settle deeper into your cushion or chair.

To allow yourself to relax fully it can help to know what you brought along with you. Try to remember your day today and how you felt:
   – how did you get up this morning?
   – did you look forward to today?
   – what was important for you in the events of the day?
        – has anything annoyed you?
        – has anything pleased you?
        – was the day peaceful or rushed?
        – what did you feel on the way to this class?

   Retrace your way here in your mind and arrive once more in your thoughts.
        – how did you feel when you first arrived here?
        – are you open and ready for this class or is something still preventing you from being fully here?

If something is still holding you back, let yourself know how you want to deal with it. Do you want to set it aside for now or do you want to talk about it?

Breathe in deeply once more, stretch and yawn.

Open your eyes again and come back into this group.

*[Breathe in and out deeply and audibly] This is meant as a comment for you as the antenatal teacher. It is important to remind *yourself* to breathe and to let go of any accumulated tension with an audible outbreath. When participants hear you 'sighing' in between it is an encouragement for them too, to breathe out and to let go of tension that built up unnoticed – until they feel it melting away, when they breathe out deeply.

Clarification of expectations

EXERCISE

POSTER

Before the first people arrive, hang four large sheets of paper on the wall, on each of which you have started a sentence:

I hope, in this antenatal class we will . . .
I hope, in this antenatal class we won't . . .
It will be a good course, if . . .
I hope we will learn something about . . .

Keep lots of felt-tip pens and encouragement ready so that everybody can finish the sentences in their own way while waiting for the others to arrive.

EXERCISE

VARIATION

Hand out a sheet of paper to everybody with the started sentences and ask the participants to finish them. Collect the sheets and, after the introduction round, write them out on a large poster yourself. That way the statements remain completely anonymous.

EXERCISE

SNOWBALL

Duration: 15 min.

This exercise is especially suited to eliciting expectation from group participants without pressure to speak in the large group. Further, it enables the participants to get to know each other better. You could suggest that women get together (first as a pair, then in a group of four or six) and that men get together for this exercise. This will automatically yield male and female expectations.

Reflect quietly on what you want and expect from this course, from the group, the group leader.

Now, write it down in one sentence.

Everybody then find a partner and share your expectations.

Together formulate a new sentence that incorporates both of your expectations. It is important that both of you should feel satisfied that the sentence expresses your individual needs.

Each pair then get together with another pair and all four of you try to find a new formulation that contains all of your individual expectations.

Each group of four then present your statement of expectations to the group.

as a group leader you can respond to the different statements with:

○ 'Yes we will do that . . .
○ I don't think it will be possible to go as far as that in the short time we have together . . .
○ This is exactly what I had in mind too . . .
○ I don't feel that I am able to give you that . . ., but I can suggest a book where you could find more information . . .' etc.

depending on what is right for you and this group. With this you establish a contract with the participants which you can refer to in future sessions.

The following illustration of course contents can be used to classify and expand the expressed expectations.

Loft
Extras, tips and exchange about nappies, layette, prams, secondhand baby gear etc.

Nursery	**Bedroom**	**Bathroom**
* Needs of the newborn child	* Relaxation	* Bodycare, tips for 'minor' ailments (teeth and gums, piles, varicose veins, cramps, backache, stretch marks)
* Needs of other children	* Breathing	
* Needs of the parents	* Birth positions	
* Our roles as father and mother	* Stretching exercises	
* Clarifying practical issues of living as a family	* Massage	* Preparation of breasts and pelvic floor
	* Sex	

Kitchen	**Lounge**	**Study**
* Nutrition during pregnancy	* Preparation for parenthood	* Information about natural birth process possible deviations and complications
* Nutrition during breastfeeding	* Communication skills (expressing needs, wishes and negations towards childbirth professionals and partner)	* Information about medical interventions (its uses and disadvantages)
* Herbal teas and . . .		
* Alternative remedies	* Discussion and exchange within the group	* Information about research, current practises etc

Foundation
Expectations, fears and other feelings as woman or man
Relationship to myself to my own body
Life experience to date
Experience with pain and stress
Emotional issues that will support or undermine the birth experience

EXERCISE

DRAWING A COURSE HOUSE

You could draw *your* own house with *your* contents, and decide how big is which room in your course house? Cut the rooms out of cardboard and 'build' the house in the group, as you refer to the expectations which you elicited from the group participants, through 'Poster' or 'Snowball' or any other method. Or show them your house model first and then ask them all to draw their houses. How big would they want the kitchen, bathroom, lounge etc. to be? That is, how much space do they want the various issues to occupy in this antenatal class? They might well come up with other rooms too. (See appendix, 'Setting your house in order', a metaphorical exercise.)

Suggestions for dealing with certain issues

EXERCISE

FLASHLIGHT

Duration: 1 min. per participant.

This exercise conveys the general atmosphere of a group very well. You can use it if you want a brief feedback, whenever you have lost touch with where the group is, or when you feel that there has been too much focus on just a few participants and you want everybody to get involved again.

Everybody can ask, at any time, for a 'flashlight' on a certain issue — particularly when it is important for the group leader or any participant to hear the point of view of all other group members on a specific theme.

The person requesting the flashlight begins by stating her own point of view or feeling; if a climate of feeling is sought, then everybody speaks up in turn.

Everybody should say something even if it is only: 'I don't want to contribute anything to this.'

Whatever is expressed in the flashlight remains 'private property'; it is not to be challenged or analysed by anybody. Nobody is allowed to come back with 'but you said . . .'.

PAIR EXERCISE

ROSARY

Duration: 2 min. to find a partner; 5 min. per person; 12 min. in total.

Two participants, A and B sit opposite each other, hold eye contact and body contact, if wanted.

Start a sentence with: 'I fear that . . .'; 'I would like to be able to . . .'; 'I would like you to . . .'; 'An ideal father/mother . . .' etc.

A begins by completing the sentence and then starting the same sentence again, completing it with a different ending, and so on.

A explores different statements all with the same sentence beginning.

B listens for 5 min. without contradicting or agreeing to anything A says.

Then without discussion they change over and B repeats the same sentence over and over again adding a different ending each time.

After both have had their turn, they can speak briefly about their experience with each other.

Conclude with a 'Flashlight' so that everyone can briefly say how s/he feels after this exercise, and what was important about what s/he or the partner said.

Variation

Work as a pair on the sentence for 5 min.

Each, alternately, completing the given sentence; or each asking the same question to the other alternately (see the following exercise).

PAIR EXERCISE

QUESTIONING

Duration: 15 min. (including finding a partner).

The exercise enables participants to look at an issue from different angles and encourages them to find the answers to important questions.

A and B sit opposite each other and maintain eye contact; body contact if wanted.

B begins to ask the given question 'How do you visualize the birth of your child?'

A answers and B listens attentively. Whenever A loses the thread or finishes, B asks the same question again, possibly in different intonations:

How do you visualize the birth of your child?
How do *you* visualize the birth of your child?
How do you visualize the *birth* of your child?
How do you visualize the birth of *your* child?

After about 7 min. (without discussion) A and B change places: A asks and B answers the questions.

You might want to conclude this questioning with a 'Flashlight' to find out what the participants discovered about themselves, where they encountered difficulties and how they felt about the exercise. You can also suggest any question that suits an issue which you want to introduce, or which was brought up by a participant: '*What* are *you* looking *forward* to?' '*How* will *your child* fit into *your* life?' '*What frightens you*?'

Depending on the question, it can be more effective if the couple does the questioning with each other, or if you suggest that women work with women and men with men.

EXERCISE

WOMEN'S GROUP/MEN'S GROUP

Duration: per theme 10–15 min. Groups work parallel to each other. Exchange of results another 10 min.

Sex-specific groups help members to focus on themselves, especially when it comes to issues that are role-fixed or particularly sensitive or personal. Further, the relative anonymity allows members to communicate difficult issues to their partners.

All members of the sex-specific group contribute their points of view to the given theme. Contributions will be recorded anonymously in writing.

Prepare and then present a statement to the other group(s).

Each group discuss the statements of the other(s) and deliver a commentary.

Possible themes

Sexuality
  – how has pregnancy altered the women's and men's view of themselves as sexual beings and their view of their partner?

Birth
  – what is the significance of this birth?

Parenthood
  – how can we help one another in this new job?

EXERCISE

SMALL GROUPS

Small groups comprise 3–7 people (depending on size of large group) and mixed sexes; partners work in different groups.

Small group work is important. As group leader you can create some breathing space for the next steps you want to take with the group as a whole, or to get clear about the issue that came up yourself. It gives the participants a chance to get to know each other better and is less inhibiting than large groups. Remember, the task must be clearly defined, it is not enough just to raise an issue and to then suggest discussion; it is important to give clear instructions (see rules above).

Further, a complex theme has to be structured. You could supply handouts or provide an example which can be copied. (Diagram to be filled in or set of questions.)
Not only are better results obtained by providing a structure, the participants also are much more able to contribute, even with potentially embarrassing themes.
As with all the other issues it becomes very clear that there is no one right answer that suits everybody. There are differing expectations and so there are different results. Whether it is methods of birth control, breathing, positions, medical help, or whatever. But you can make a better choice if you know what your expectations and attitudes are. Also your expectations and attitudes might change as you share them with other people.

Duration: 10–20 min. depending on scope of the given theme.

All participants of the small group contribute their own points of view and experience. Discuss findings.

One person from the small group note down the findings or collected points of views, and present them afterwards to the large group.

The group leader should remind the small groups of the task half way through the allotted time. (It is very easy to 'branch off' during small group discussions, and avoid dealing with the selected theme.)

The group leader should remind the small groups of the time 3 min. before the end of the allotted time so that they have a chance of finalizing their statement, or collection of experiences, answers, or whatever is asked of them.

Conclude with a large group discussion or a 'Flashlight.'

Possible themes:

Likes and dislikes of pregnancy so far.

Knowledge of breastfeeding and sources of information.

Mistakes and benefits in our own upbringing.

Example of structuring the task

What I learned about birth and pregnancy as a child	What I think about it now	What made me change my mind
....	....	....
....	....	....

Even giving a clearly defined theme such as: 'The method of birth control you find most suitable', is still too complex. The participants themselves are probably not clear about it and would rather get more information from the group leader. It is usually a participant who asks the antenatal teacher which method of birth control would she recommend for after the baby is born. In order for participants to find the answer for themselves, you, the group leader, could prepare 10 or 12 small cards (one set for each small group) on which aspects of birth control have been noted; for example:

  – safe as possible
  – no hormonal interference
  – easy to use
  – easy to obtain
  – no regular medical check-ups necessary
  – not to interfere with breastfeeding
  – not messy
  – not only the woman's responsibility
  – least side-effects
  – inexpensive
  – no fiddling that might be a turn off
  – no interruption of sexual togetherness

The task for the small groups is to choose 4 of these 10 cards — i.e. to choose four aspects that each participant in his/her small group can agree on as being the most important. Certain methods of birth control are eliminated automatically in the process, so the group is able to bring at least part results into the large group.

EXERCISE

INFORMATION WASHING LINE

Hang a string, with clothes pegs on it, so that after each small group session 'results' can be displayed for everybody to read during a later break.

Silent reflection

Not everything has to be expressed or talked about; often silent reflection is just as effective. Have pens and paper ready so that participants can make notes on whichever theme you want them to think about.

EXERCISE

┌─ **BRAINSTORMING** ──────────────────────────

Write down any association (word, phrase, symbol or image) to a certain word. For example: 'birth', 'labour ward', 'pain', 'baby', 'breast' etc., whatever the theme is that you want to introduce or structure (see page 189).

EXERCISE

┌─ **DRAWING UP A LIST** ──────────────────────

Using one of the following sets of questions, everyone can draw up his/her own list. These can function as a lead in to group discussion or as a stimulus to further thought and discussion outside the group.

○ – which medical intervention would I accept if necessary?
....
....

– which medical interventions do I want to avoid at all costs?
....
....

○ – who or what do I trust?
....
....

– who or what do I distrust?
....
....

○ – what can I give my child?
....
....

– what do I want to give my child?
....
....

○ – positive aspects of pregnancy
....
....

– negative aspects of pregnancy
....
....

EXERCISE

WRITING A CREDO _____

Ask participants to:
'Write down your own beliefs, "articles of faith" to a certain
theme; everything that comes to mind. You can distinguish later
whether what you wrote down is nonsense, outdated or still
acceptable to you.'

For example
   I believe men are . . .
   I believe women are . . .
   I believe children need . . .
   I believe birth is . . .
   etc.

Encouraging the group to express themselves

EXERCISE

PLEBISCITO _____

○ *Eliciting participants' preferences*
Using a large sheet of paper, prepare a list, for example of
things the partners can do to help at birth.

Hand out 5 sticky dots, different colours for men and women.
Ask participants to pinpoint the suggestions they would most
like to follow. Having to make a choice helps participants to
focus on their preferences. It creates a graphic display of where
the group as a whole is at.

Alternately different interventions can be listed and two sets of
3 sticky dots can be handed out to everybody. To point out the
most (green) and least favoured (red) intervention.

○ *For feedback*

Everybody gets stickers of two different colours (for example:
red for negative feedback; green for positive feedback).
List all the items, main exercises and issues that have featured
in the course so far, and ask the participants to give one
coloured dot to the item(s) they are satisfied with and another
coloured dot to the item(s) they are not satisfied with. This
method is also useful at the beginning of a course to elicit
participants' expectations. Everybody gets five dots and can
stick them to the item on the list that seems most important to
them.

Example:
(*ten participants distributing five dots each*)

Getting to know other couples	**
Film/slideshow about birth	***
Medical information	********
Gymnastics	**
Breastfeeding	*****

Pregnancy and sexuality	*
Caring for a newborn baby	**
Preparation for life as a family	*
Breathing	*********
Bodycare	*
Fatherhood . . . Motherhood . . .	**
Relaxation	******
Birth positions	*
Birth process	***
Dealing with fear	
Home birth versus hospital birth	**
Legal issues	
Experiencing the child within	**

EXERCISE

USING SYMBOLIC PICTURES

Whenever you find a specially pleasing, annoying or symbolically meaningful picture in a magazine or newspaper ad. cut it out and stick it on a piece of cardboard. There are various uses for them.

At the first session participants could choose one of the pictures to introduce themselves ('This is how I feel at the moment' or 'This picture is meaningful to me because . . .'). It might be an image of a waterfall, a flower meadow, a gypsy caravan or a modern motor home, a flashy sports car, a detailed and complex bit of machinery, a worn out woman or man sitting on the roadside, a lively festivity going on or the lonely back of a person on a hillside, etc. The more images you collect the greater the choice. Ideally you should have at least two per participant. You could use these cardboard pictures too, to work on certain issues. The small groups (3–4 participants) should choose from a choice of 10 images the one they feel represents most what 'Fatherhood' means to them, or 'Motherhood', 'Childhood', 'Sexuality', 'Birth', whatever theme you would like to explore with this method.

EXERCISE

WAILING WOMEN

Sometimes it is impossible to work on a certain theme, because there seem to be so many complaints being voiced — the cramps, the fatigue, the lack of understanding of partner, parents, colleagues, the hospital situation and so on. Sometimes so many complaints and disappointments are present that there is little energy left to focus forward. But instead of suppressing such feelings, it is better to encourage them to come out. Everybody should talk, complain, groan, moan, yammer, wail at the same time. The importance is not so much to be listened to, as to get it out! The complaining lasts for as long as it takes and usually ends when the emotional release brings about refreshed perspectives and a good laugh about ourselves. In good time, focus again on the theme of the session.

EXERCISE

TEXT PUZZLE

Choose an aphorism, a sentence or saying that is in close connection with the theme you want to explore with the class. Write it in individual words on pieces of cardboard. The sentence should contain as many words as there are participants in the group. Every participant is given one word.

The group tries to build a sentence out of its puzzle pieces.

For the first 3–5 min. each person is only allowed to put down and remove their own word. They should not speak with each other, give hints to others or discuss what the sentence might be.

In the second phase each person is allowed to remove the word card of another person *once* and place it somewhere else, still not speaking.

In the third phase participants can talk with each other and try to figure out the sentence by discussing it.

Examples:

| Practice | is | mechanical | and | always | removes | you |
| from | what | is | | | | (10) |

| The | essence | of | creativity | is | an | aware |
| balance | between | control | and | surrender | | (12) |

True	freedom	means	no	internal	choice –	the
seed	contains	within	it	its	demand	for	action
							(15)

| The | mystery | of | life | is | not | a | problem | to | be |
| solved | but | a | reality | to | be | experienced | | | (17) |

The	future	is	virgin	territory,	planted	by	my
feelings	and	thoughts	in	the	present,	nothing
can	exist	in	the	future	that	I	do	not	want
to	be	there.

(28 words, yes it is possible in fairly large groups too).

This is a good way to introduce a reflection or discussion about fairly philosophical concepts. The group will be much more able to discuss an abstract concept once they have created the sentence themselves

EXERCISE

> ## FOUR CORNERS
>
> Four large sheets of paper, each with a different question or challenging statement, are placed in each corner of the room.
>
> The participants are invited to gather in the corner with the question or statement they would most like to discuss. The small groups that assemble in this way then discuss why they chose this particular corner/question (Maybe because the question is their own question or because they know a clear answer to it; maybe because they disagree with it vehemently or because they support it fully). Proceed as with 'small groups' (page 175).

EXERCISE

> ## CASE WORK
>
> Gather in small groups.
>
> Each small group receives the same 'Case', a specific conflict situation in the context of pregnancy, birth or parenthood.
>
> Discuss within a given time a solution for this problem.
>
> Now contribute your solution(s) to the large group.
>
> Often several possible solutions are apparent; which is an important experience; there is not one right solution for each case.
>
> The group leader might want to prepare a few cases to have available.
>
> Someone may have a story to tell — which lends itself to scrutiny by the group in small groups.

Role play as method

This is a valuable tool with which to explore future roles.

To help overcome the common resistance to role play, give clear instructions and make it clear no one is watching.

Ask the participants to gather in small groups, all role play simultaneously. It is not important to be seen in one's role, but to experience it oneself.

EXERCISE

┌─ **SITCOM** ──────────────────────────────────────

The players receive a description of a situation; for example:

> Sunday afternoon. Aunt/sister/mother/friend is visiting. They all sit around on the sofa etc. Wife breastfeeding the baby, chatting with Aunt; husband reading the Sunday papers; baby falls asleep at the breast. After 10 minutes the baby wakes up again and starts crying. The aunt takes the baby out of the mother's arms and rocks him saying 'My poor little soul, you're still hungry are you? They don't give you enough, do they? Shall I make you a lovely bowl of cereal?'

The three players take the scene from here. How will the mother, the father react? How will the conversation or argument develop? The participants play themselves according to their feelings about breastfeeding or they can choose an exaggerated attitude and explore how they feel in play acting this role. You can suggest that men try playing mother and women try playing father; this often helps participants to understand the other part better.

EXERCISE

┌─ **IMPROVISATION** ─────────────────────────────────

Each small group receives small cards which contain a word or term that should set no more than an impetus.

For example, a pink card: First visit to cinema after the birth, and four green cards: mother, father, friend, baby-sitter, or pink card: Smoking aunt/uncle arrives in non-smoking household with newborn baby; green cards: mother, father, uncle/aunt, friend; or pink card: Baby demands breastfeeding in cafe; green cards: mother, father, waiter, waitress, manager

From these few words the small group should develop a short play.

EXERCISE

┌─ **A-B-C ROLE PLAY** ───────────────────────────────

The large group divides into small groups of 3 members each. In each small group they decide who is A (father), who is B (mother), who is C (friend).

The special feature of this method of role play is that in each small group there are always two players and one observer. Three scenarios are played, each lasting about 3 min. As group leader you can either hand out a sheet containing the information to each small group, or prepare a poster for all (see following description). After the role play talk about the experiences felt in the large group ('flashlight' or group discussion).

Theme: Role expectation

A = Father   B = Mother   C = Friend

1st set (C = Observer)

Father stands at the changing mat, cooing with little baby. After a while mother enters and notices that the nappy doesn't fit properly. She exclaims: 'For heaven's sake, why can't you learn how to fit a nappy properly? Look how loose that is, she will be wet all over in no time.'
Play on from there for about 3 min. then exchange observations for about 2 min.

2nd set (A = Observer)

Mother meets her friend at the street corner. They start chatting and the friend says to the mother: 'You know what I really like about your husband, he is so helpful at home, he even changes nappies.'
Play on from there for about 3 min. then exchange observations for about 2 min.

3rd set (B = Observer)

Friend visits and finds husband in the kitchen making tea for everybody. He sighs: 'You know I don't think I'm really valued around here.'
Play on from here for about 3 min., then exchange observations for about 2 min.

The observer observes only and does not interact in the play or pass comment. After each set the players exchange feelings on how they experienced themselves, and each other, and then the observer adds what he or she noticed as an 'outsider'.

EXERCISE

EVALUATION OF THE ROLE PLAY

Make sure there is always enough time left to evaluate the role playing. Introduce questions to help the participants reflect further on their own role playing.
- did you experience yourself as behaving realistically in your roles?
- what made you choose a certain role?
- did you choose roles that were easy for you or did you explore with a role that seemed difficult to you?
- which of your personal attitudes, motifs, peculiarities, did you re-discover in your role?

- which solutions were found in the different role plays?
- what was the actual difference in the outcome of the various small groups. What led to the different solutions?
- which arguments were decisive? What did you learn?

It is what one learns about oneself that is important in the evaluation, not the playing itself. Usually many clichés are expressed in the role play and it is worth while reflecting:
- where do clichés come from? i.e. the lazy man, the over-anxious wife, the bossy mother-in-law.
- why is it easier to make fun of clichés, exaggerating them, rather than trying out new modes of behaviour?
- what happened when men played the role of a woman, or women played the role of a man?

And lastly the most important question:
- what role does the child play, while the parents are involved in their role-conflict?

Using film or slides

Luckily there is no perfect film or slide show when it comes to showing birth. Most films cause frequent dissatisfaction, and raise questions. So take courage, even the showing of a mediocre or bad film (if you have the facilities, and the group expresses interest) can be used.

It is exactly the faults the film or slide-show might have (showing unfavourable position, breathing, handling of the delivery etc.) that are a bonus. Nobody can sit back and say how wonderful, but you can raise all the questionable parts if the group doesn't do it by themselves, and get a discussion going.

As with all the methods suggested here, the method is only a means to an end. It is the discussion and the exchange of thoughts that follow which are important. No method is ultimately better than another. It is your individual choice, making sure it suits your style and the needs of this particular group, that makes a method good.

Different methods for eliciting feedback

It is useful to ask for feedback halfway through the course rather than at the end; after all, there is more point in knowing when something can still be done about it. Accordingly, you might want to establish a new contract with the group, point out boundaries or change your course plan.

At the last session you could make a guided tour with the participants, leading them briefly through the whole course once more. From the beginning, how they arrived, the various main exercises you did, the various themes and issues you covered (all in the rough order of how it took place), to where they are 'at' now. You can remind them of controversial issues that came up and/or certain solutions you might have found in the course of the class. Do this slowly with pauses so that images and memories can come up. After the 'guided fantasy' ask for a 'flashlight' where everybody can say what they had difficulties remembering or connecting to, what sprang to mind most easily and what had been the most important event for them in the course of the class.

Of course you can just ask for it. It depends on how aware and articulate the group is whether or not this is effective. Most people find it difficult to express dissatisfaction so you might get a false feedback.

To encourage participants to come out with negative comments too you could try the following.

EXERCISE

DARTING FEEDBACK

Draw a dartboard on a large sheet of paper and hang up. Divide it into three areas: one for exercises, one for the content, one for the group discussions. Each participant gets three sticky dots to place one into every area. The closer to the centre he or she places the dot the more satisfaction is expressed. The further away from the centre the dot gets placed the more dissatisfaction is expressed.

Variation

Hand out three different coloured buttons or cards to each participant:

green for greatest agreement, yellow for neutral, red for least agreement.

Place three white sheets in the centre of the group. On each is written, respectively, 'Information', 'Exercises', 'Group Atmosphere'.

Everybody places one card or button on each of the sheets. Only this allows for differentiated feedback even though participants might find it difficult to put down a green button if they weren't at all happy or a red button if they don't feel in any way dissatisfied. Look out for the nuances. There must be one area in which you feel a little bit more or less satisfied with, than another.

Once the dartboard or the sheets are fitted it is a lot easier for the group to express their feedback.

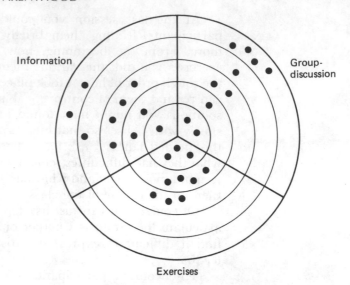

QUESTIONNAIRE

You might want to hand out a questionnaire like A at the beginning of the course for statistical information if you want those sort of facts in writing, or B at the end of the course for your own feedback.

Questionnaire A

Who or what made you interested in
coming to antenatal classes?
GP   ◯
Friend   ◯
Partner   ◯
Other?   ◯

How did you find out that and where the
classes take place?
GP (unit)   ◯
Friend   ◯
Partner   ◯
Newspaper   ◯
Poster   ◯
Other?   ◯

Where would you like to have your baby?

....

Have you made contact with the
clinic/midwife already?
Yes   ◯
No   ◯

Do you intend to breastfeed?
Maybe   ◯
No   ◯
Yes, for a few weeks   ◯
Yes, as long as possible   ◯

Would you want 'rooming in'?
Maybe   ◯
No   ◯
Complete 'rooming' in   ◯
Part 'rooming in'   ◯

Whom would you like to be present at
birth?
Midwife   ◯
Doctor   ◯
Partner   ◯
Mother   ◯
Friend   ◯
Don't know yet   ◯
Only doctor and midwife   ◯
Only midwife   ◯

Did you visit the clinic of your choice?
Yes   ○
No   ○

How old are you?
under 20   ○
20–25   ○
25–30   ○
30–35   ○
35–40   ○
over 40   ○

Will the people of your choice be able to be there?
Most likely   ○
If possible   ○
Probably not   ○
No   ○

Are you male?   ○

Are you female?   ○

Are you expecting your first baby?   ○

Do you have other children?   ○

Questionnaire B   *Feedback*

	Negative		Neutral	Positive	
	++	+		+	++
Was the information you received valuable?	○	○	○	○	○
Was the course helpful in reducing your fears?	○	○	○	○	○
Did you gain in self confidence?	○	○	○	○	○
Did you like the atmosphere in the group?	○	○	○	○	○
Did you feel free to contribute what you wanted?	○	○	○	○	○
Did you like the way the course was run?	○	○	○	○	○
Did you like the approach of your antenatal teacher?	○	○	○	○	○
How did you like the physical exercises?	○	○	○	○	○
Did you like the way breathing was taught?	○	○	○	○	○
Did you find the group discussions meaningful?	○	○	○	○	○
Did you like the relaxation exercises?	○	○	○	○	○
Did you find the course as a whole varied enough?	○	○	○	○	○
Did you find the course material used useful?	○	○	○	○	○
Did you find the course material used well designed?	○	○	○	○	○
Was the amount of course material adequate?	○	○	○	○	○
Was the number of sessions sufficient?	○	○	○	○	○
Was the length of the sessions about right?	○	○	○	○	○
Did you like the room in which the course was held?	○	○	○	○	○

Further suggestions

More time should be spent on   ....

Less time should be spent on   ....

The course should not deal with   ....

I missed the mentioning/teaching/exploring of   ....

Working with large groups

It might not always be possible to work with small groups. For whatever reasons (e.g. institutional or local pressure) your number of participants might be over 16, up to 30, or even more, which can be exhausting. Traditionally antenatal teaching in large groups has taken the form of one part devoted to a particular type of breathing, relaxation exercises and gymnastics, and another to talks given by the group leader or a guest speaker. There might be time for questions but seldom time enough for exchange of thoughts amongst the participants. Some antenatal teachers maintain that even when sufficient time is provided, the participants do not come forth readily, and there are not enough differentiated questions and no personal statements. 'All they seem to want to do *is* sit back and listen'.

But it does not need to be like that. If you want a more lively group you can use all the methods mentioned so far. You need more structure and preparation than for smaller sized groups, though. Also, as you don't have the advantage of the 'fruits' from the group process, you have to supply more input as group leader.

Some tips for working with larger groups.

- Bring yourself in as a 'person' rather than just a 'professional'. Participants will only open up when they experience *you* as open. Share something from your life situation, your personal birth experience etc.
- Offer information in such a way that participants can connect it to their own experience. Only then can the received information be used.
- Offer plenty of opportunity for exploring attitudes, beliefs, feelings, likes and dislikes.
- Offer possibilities for trying out new and different modes of behaviour. Big changes finally come about only following lots of little changes.
- Offer plenty of controversial themes to provoke thought and discussion but avoid any interpretation as 'right' or 'wrong'.
- Limit any teacher-talking time to less than 10 minutes.
- Limit open group discussion by introducing a method or exercise as soon as you feel the thread is getting lost.

There really need not be that much difference between a large group and a regular sized group (the main difference you will feel is in your own exhaustion and that is the main point that speaks against working with large groups). But before you let yourself be persuaded to work with large groups in the above mentioned sense ask yourself:
  – do I believe that the experience and knowledge of the participant is of equal value to mine and do I use that insight in my work?
  – how important do I find the interaction between the participants and between the participants and myself?

23 Ways of dealing with specific topics

Dealing with pain

Ask participants to note the associations that the word 'pain' brings up and to reflect on their significance with one of the following.

EXERCISE

GROUP EXERCISE WITH BALL

Sit in a circle.

Whenever someone throws the ball, he or she says the word 'pain'.

Whoever receives the ball must say whatever word immediately comes to mind.

This exercise can be done with many other words such as 'Mother-hood'/'Baby'/'Stress' etc. when working with other topics. Due to the speed of the exercise unconscious associations emerge.

Brainstorming can be a good way to approach the subject of pain in antenatal classes. It only takes a few minutes for everybody to write down their own associations and then to share them with the rest of the group. The sharing can be particularly valuable as associations may be offered that had not occurred to everybody but make sense when suggested. You can add things which had not been mentioned – for example 'separation' may not have been associated with pain. Simply identifying and sharing associations are meaningful in themselves so that people can identify and evaluate their beliefs. Interpretation is not usually needed.

EXERCISE

BRAINSTORMING

Each person makes a list of words, phrases, symbols etc. that come to mind with the word 'pain'. A couple of volunteers read their lists out to the others who can add their own associations. These can then be collected on the board. The course leader can take the opportunity to bring out the inner connections between various contributions or to point out any one-sidedness in the contributions as a whole. See next page.

Example: Association to pain

Fight/Defend against
Conquer/Succumb to
Suppress
Control
Judge/Condemn
Make light of/Trivialize
Accept/Acknowledge
Overcome/Be overcome by

Power – my body's power over me
      – the power over others that
        being in pain gives me

Needing or wanting pain
      – to receive sympathy
      – to be able to accept love
      – to obtain care

Inability to accept help/love/care

Fear of losing self-control,
Fear of 'making a scene'

Signal – that something is wrong
      – that there is something (else)
        I need

These are key ideas to attend to and to bring up yourself if nobody else does

Waiting	Yearning	Damage	Separation
Patience	Helplessness	Medication	Change
Suffering	Anger	Sweating	Loss
Letting go	Confusion	Vomiting	Departure
	Loneliness	Nausea	Death
	Darkness	Cold and heat	Desolation
	Challenge	Shaking	

The next step is to discover what can help to soothe and ease the pain of labour. If time is short you can summarize the various techniques and approaches or introduce or repeat the stress sequence (see page 122) so that the participants can experience what actually helps them to deal with pain. The group can then identify and share the ways in which pain can be eased. If the latter approach is used it is always helpful to finish by offering a concise summary, as not everyone is able to pick out and remember the salient points from a wide ranging discussion.

Some suggestions for coping with pain in labour

Mental strategies

○ *Understanding* mechanics of the birth process
  – the onset and stages of labour.
  – what happens to mother, what happens to baby.

○ *Accepting* labour as normal and natural
  – muscles hurt when they are working hard
  – pain is a signal: here is the action; send me your energy, your oxygen
  – the baby's descent through the birth canal causes pressure and stretching.

○ *Being aware* of the time span
  – of each contraction and of labour as a whole.

○ *Concentrating* on something positive
  – welcome each contraction as bringing the birth one step nearer.
  – remember that your child is being born
  – visualize the baby descending and rotating
  – visualize your cervix opening
  – visualize a river, growing wider and stronger*
  – visualize walking through a corridor with a series of doors that open automatically as you approach
  – visualize climbing a mountain
  – visualize surfing on waves
  – visualize walking down a long dark tunnel; focus on the ever-enlarging light at the end
  – focus on flowers or a plant in the room
  – concentrate on a favourite picture, piece of music or scent (e.g. aromatherapy oil or incense)

Physical strategies

○ *Giving* in to the demands of your body
  – relax; breathe 'naturally'
  – adopt whatever position your body dictates
  – flow with the contraction

○ *Letting go* and surrender
  – relinquish any unnatural composed behaviour (e.g. the need to make polite/witty conversation)

○ *Moving with* the pain
  – walk, sway, rock your pelvis back and forth

*It is of questionable value to offer images like a pleasant garden, a gentle stream or a flower opening its petals. Most women find that they don't match their birth experience, but lead to disappointment and a sense of failure.

Partner's strategies

○ *Giving love, emotional and physical attention and comfort*
  – offer drinks, warmth, cushions
  – offer something to suck or bite on
  – offer a moist sponge for refreshing
  – give encouragement
  – share the experience of pain, let her squeeze you or hold you tight
  – praise her with your eyes, scared, worried or disgusted looking eyes betray verbal compliments and encouragement
  – offer general massage to aid relaxation and local touch relaxation to ease specific foci of pain

Give couples the space and encouragement to discuss and then try out and experiment with techniques. In this way they can identify what their own specific needs might be and gain confidence and trust in their own resources and abilities. You might want to repeat or introduce some massage and touch relaxation in this context (see page 143). This could be followed by a discussion on the stress of labour and on the uses, advantages and disadvantages of the various pain relieving drugs available for labour. You can also include a guided fantasy.

EXERCISE

GUIDED FANTASY: PAIN IN LABOUR

Before using the guided fantasy it is important that you write your own script, using your own words and phrases so that it feels right to you and appropriate for the people you are teaching.

Imagine that labour has started.

Contractions have begun.

How do you imagine they will feel?

How do you think you will react?

Now imagine that the contractions are getting stronger and more painful than you expected . . .

What is your fantasy of how you will cope with them?

Can you (the woman) imagine accepting the pain as a normal and natural part of letting go and giving birth to your baby?

Do you think you would choose to have medication to help nullify the pain so you can cope better and relax?

How would you feel?

What would you want to do?

What would you want from your partner?

What do you (the partner) think you will feel when your partner is in pain?

Can you imagine just being there, unable to help?

What do you feel you would want to do?

How would you like to react?

What would you like your partner to do ?

What do you think you will need for yourself?

It is important to allow enough time for people to assimilate what they have experienced and, if they choose to, to be able to share it with the group. The teacher can encourage partners to talk to each other about their fantasies and their expectations of themselves and of each other.

The localization of the pain is often meaningful. The pain is usually felt there, where most of the changes/actions take place: the back, the lower abdomen, the perineum. So the pain is a signal to us, here is the action, send me your energy, your oxygen, your warmth, your massage. The body is helping us to help it.

It is important though not to get stuck with the word pain when you talk about labour. While it is important not to pretend there is no pain or discomfort, the focus should always be brought back to the words *labour, work, effort*: There is no really strenuous effort that isn't painful. The pain of childbirth is not the pain of sickness or injury, but of work.

Muscles hurt when doing hours of strenuous exercise, be it running a marathon, chopping wood or giving birth.

So it is not just important to look at what pain means to us, but also to explore what strain and stress mean to us.

○ Try to remember a specific situation in your life that was stressful for you. It might have been a stressful period at work or mountaineering.
○ Remember how you coped with it at the time? What was most difficult about it? What kept you going?
○ Let yourself know whether you are a type of person who quite enjoys stressful situations — the challenge, the extra adrenalin that goes with it — or whether you tend to avoid any stress if you can help it.

If there is a lot of energy (need) in a particular group about the issues of pain or stress you might want to introduce:

EXERCISE

A PAIR EXERCISE TO EXPLORE OUR REACTION TO PAIN OR STRESS

> – Find a partner. One person talks for 5 minutes, the other person listens, if necessary helps with question but no comment or contribution at that point. After 5 minutes, change over and the other person gets a chance to talk while the first person listens.
> – Each describe three situations in your life that were painful/stressful and talk about how you dealt with them.
> 1. Situation as a child
> 2. Situation as an adolescent
> 3. Situation as an adult
>
> Who or what was helpful at the time? What was your reaction to those situations? What did you learn from them. After the exercise you can suggest a Flashlight on the questions: What did you discover about yourself? Can you recognize a certain pattern of behaviour in yourself. Was there a change in your behaviour over the years?

It is not only valuable to encourage the participants in antenatal classes to reflect on their own pattern of reaction to stress or pain, but to point out that everybody reacts differently, that there is no right or wrong and to acknowledge the differences within the relationship. The patterns of behaviour of man and wife are often different, so it is helpful to the pair to respect each other's reactions rather than holding wrong expectations.

Dealing with fear

Fear increases our general level of arousal and alerts our protective mechanisms. Generally, this is a positive, motivating factor, propelling people to make changes in their lives. In the context of pregnancy and childbirth preparations this may involve a review of the place or circumstances of the birth, and talking through wishes with professionals, as well as making practical arrangements for good support and help after the birth. In the context of the birth itself however, even the smallest amount of fear affects the hormonal flow, makes us physically and emotionally tense and can inhibit the birthing process. But it is natural to fear the unknown and for many women giving birth is an unknown; even if they've had a baby before and so are familiar with the mechanics of birth. A second or subsequent labour may be entirely different. So, while fear or at least apprehension is a natural feature of approaching labour, it is still a valuable exercise to identify any rational or irrational fears and attempt to deal with them. The irrational fears, in particular, can wreak havoc and so should either be understood and accepted or eliminated so that precious labouring energy is not wasted in fighting it.

Giving full and accurate information can help to allay irrational fears by providing perspective and the proper context. Tell participants in class that acknowledging and being open about their fears will help towards an easier birth and transition to parenthood. Often, participants feel guilty about harming the baby with their anxiety, which might make them feel isolated and 'abnormal.'

So, sharing fears and worries can in itself lighten the load. Any of the following exercises is suitable for either introducing or structuring the theme once it comes up spontaneously. Somebody in the group might talk about their fear and, to relieve the focus on that one person, you want to take the theme up for the whole group; or you might sense a lot of unconscious and suppressed fear in a particular group and work on from there.

If there is really no fear 'around' you don't need to spend much time on it. But do talk about it briefly mentioning its positive sides too, and the importance of acknowledging fears.

Sometimes *you* might feel it is necessary for the group, yet the group resists to follow up the exercise you suggested. It is better not to give in ('Alright let's do something else instead'), and to continue with breathing, massage, or whatever the next 'topic' is, but to suggest 'Let's just try it for 2 minutes if the 5 minutes seem daunting to you'. There is always an unpleasant feeling left if one leaves a subject unexplored, however well one can rationalize it!

Sometimes participants are so afraid of their own fear that they don't use the pair exercise in the way you suggest but talk about something else. But that's alright too: it is important to offer and suggest but not to push. Everyone has his/her own boundaries and self-protective resistance and they can't be broken by mere suggestion unless the person wants them broken. Nobody will feel fear that wasn't there anyway. Nobody will start crying unless he or she was ready for it and just needed a trigger.

On the other hand you can help the participants to 'get to grips' with the theme by allowing them to theorize about it.

You have to be clear in your own mind what you want to offer at a certain moment. Trust your instinct, whether you feel safe and at ease with it. The group will notice if you introduce the exercise with insecurity. If you are not sure about it, leave it.

There is always the possibility for you, too, to share your fears with the group. You are working with a group of mature intelligent people.

EXERCISE

QUESTIONING IN PAIRS (see page 173) ON FEAR

This exercise is more effective if couples don't work together. Encourage the formation of woman–woman, man–man pairs.

A asks:

What do *you fear* when *you* think about the *birth* of *your child*?

The question is asked several times with varying intonation.

B answers the question within the allocated 5 min.

Now B asks the question with varying intonation and A answers.

EXERCISE

ROSARY (see page 173) ON FEAR

Working in pairs of the same sex, each in turn completes one of the following sentences:

I fear that . . .
My fear is that . . .
I'm afraid of . . .

Allocate 5 min. per person.

EXERCISE

WOMEN'S GROUP/MEN'S GROUP (see page 174) ON FEAR

Each group gathers and notes down on a large sheet of paper all the fears they have about pregnancy, birth and/or parenthood. Allow 10–20 min. 'Post' the findings on the wall (or on an 'info. washing line') for all to peruse.

EXERCISE

PLEBISCITO (see page 178) ON FEAR

Divide group into men and women.

Prepare two posters listing many fears:

dying during labour/at delivery
baby dying
baby malformed
baby mentally handicapped
baby physically handicapped
complications at birth

needing drugs
baby needing intensive care
caesarean delivery
forceps delivery
episiotomy
baby presenting breech
not reaching hospital in time
midwife/doctor not arriving on time
partner being held up
unpleasant midwife
intolerable pain

Groups to put one sticky dot per member on those points members are most afraid of; limit the number of dots to 5 per member.

Whichever exercise you use, there is usually a distinction between women's and men's fears regarding childbirth (or parenthood, if that's your theme). And that fact alone gets a discussion going.

You can introduce the distinction between panic and fear. You can talk about the positive aspects of fear.

Fear of postnatal depression

The notion of postnatal depression – and with it the fear of it – is a popular one and has been around for a very long time. In nearly every class there will be a woman, or couple, who have had a neighbour or friend who felt 'depressed' or disappointed after their baby was born and will therefore be afraid of it, even if the fear is not often expressed openly.

I believe it is important for antenatal teachers to stress to couples in class the difference between the popular notion of so-called postnatal depression, i.e. a woman *feeling* low as part of a natural process of readjustment, and the clinical condition, i.e. a woman actually *being* depressed and therefore being unable to cope with motherhood. Only a very small number of women suffer from clinical postnatal depression, and they need proper medical attention, whereas most women will feel disappointed, ambivalent, stressed or 'depressed' at some point or other after birth as a natural result of the fundamental changes taking place in their bodies and their lives, just as they would or could following other momentous changes in their lives.

The birth of a child is one of the most fundamental changes in a woman's life, affecting her body as well as her image of herself, and it is therefore helpful for couples in class to be reminded of all the changes to be expected and prepared for.

The physical changes include:

○ uterus and abdominal muscles receding, often contracting painfully

○ discharge of blood from the uterus, sometimes leading to soreness

○ engorged breasts and sore or even very painful nipples if cracked

○ intestines readjusting to space vacated, perhaps resulting in constipation or painful motions

○ bladder readjusting to new space, possibly making it more difficult to feel the need to pass urine

○ pelvic floor weakened, occasionally giving rise to stress incontinence

○ perineum still sore or even very painful while a tear, cut or bruise is healing

○ heart and blood circulation readjusting to less blood to be supplied

Quite apart from these aches and pains enough to make any woman feel weak, weepy and uncomfortable, all these physical changes take energy out of the body. Yet, a woman cannot just rest and take care of herself, because there is the baby to feed or to comfort, to change or to settle – day and night, without break, disrupting the normal sleep pattern. It is not surprising that the woman feels fatigue and often a sense of inadequacy, particularly if the baby is not easily consoled, and as she gets no break from her responsibility of caring for the baby's needs, it is not uncommon or unnatural for an exasperated, overtired mother not to feel loving towards the baby, but more like putting a pillow over her screaming child's face or even catch herself thinking of throwing the baby out of the window.

These feelings are also caused or intensified by the rapid changes in the hormone balance after birth. During pregnancy, the hormone progesterone acts as a natural tranquillizer, as a result of which some women feel better than ever during pregnancy. For instance, research has shown that no psychotic states occur in women during pregnancy, not even in women that would otherwise be prone to them. Before birth, an extra large amount of progesterone is produced to help with the stress of birth, but once the placenta has been delivered, the woman is suddenly deprived of her progesterone production, nature's 'tranquillizer'.

Apart from these mainly physical processes, there are the psychological changes and influences a woman is subject to. The media in our culture only show one side of reality, that of blissful motherhood, maternal rosiness, of mothers loving their babies and looking glamorous while doing so. In baby books, in magazines, in television adverts, in films, everywhere images of a happy, beautiful, well-groomed and dressed mother with her bonny babe abound. These images are a real burden to women and do a great disservice to all womankind. Mothers feel guilty or even cheated if they do not live up to these images. After all, the media do not show images of the much more common reality of women not getting out of their dressing gowns for weeks, of the housework not getting done, of babies crying all the time, of their partners not supporting them. So women feel that there is something wrong with them if they do not radiate with happiness and contentment, or if they do not look or feel glamorous and brim with vitality.

In a culture like ours where the myth and image of women is perpetuated who 'get up and go', who are unruffled by their periods, where pregnancy and birth are 'sanitized' in the media, an expectation is created that the birth of a child is but a minor hiccup hardly disturbing normal routine. This expectation is harmful in that it does not allow women to accept the time needed for physical, emotional and psychological readjustment to take its course after the birth of a child as a natural process and transition to be undergone, as a valuable experience to be had. For change and process to happen in a person's life, all experiences have to be accepted and dealt with, rather than resisted or hurried along, and antenatal teaching should therefore not be a sort of 'scotch guard', protecting women from any unpleasant experiences or unwanted emotions they may encounter.

There is so much to cope with. Every postnatal period contains numerous genuine reasons to be upset

Apart from the physical and psychological aspects, there are big emotional adjustments to be made in the postnatal period, coming to terms with the loss of the old self, loss of pregnancy, disappointing birth experience etc.

Contrary to expectations, a happy pregnancy, a fulfilling relationship and a competent woman do not automatically result in a happy postnatal time but often lead to a difficult period of transition. The more the pregnancy was enjoyed, the greater the loss of it. A woman may have felt closer to her baby whose movements she felt inside than she does after the birth when the baby has become a separate being, she may mourn the loss of her roundedness and fertile fullness etc. The more the couple had a fulfilled and happy relationship with each other, the greater the disruption through the baby. A couple may feel resentful at not being able to go out or entertain friends, they may long to have time for leisurely sex and uninterrupted closeness, they may be unhappy about having to share the partner with the baby etc. The more a woman enjoyed a demanding job and coped well with managing and organizing her projects, the more she may feel a failure if the birth experience did not live up to her expectations of herself or if she cannot cope with the unpredictability a baby can bring into her life.

Being prepared for all these eventualities, can help women come to terms with the less rosy reality of motherhood because they no longer need to fear that there is something wrong with them if they find themselves being weepy and unstable or if they feel they cannot cope. We no longer have the support of extended families in Western societies, and this places a greater burden on a woman and, indeed, on both partners in a couple to cope with all the pains and strains of the first few weeks after birth. Being aware of this, could help husbands or partners understand what a woman is going through during this period and how they can help themselves or reach out for help amongst relatives, friends or postnatal support groups.

Knowing that their sense of inadequacy may very well be a totally natural reaction that they share with lots of other women, being made aware that these feelings are temporary and not a permanent affliction, will help many women and allow them to communicate and share their feelings rather than hide them. Being given an opportunity to have a good night's sleep, to have time for a luxurious bath, a hairdresser's appointment, and being offered practical support and loving attention will help women feeling this normal 'reactive depression' much more than any tranquillizers. Helping them to accept their experience and to 'go with it' by encouraging them to have a positive attitude towards this time in their lives could even allow women to feel special for what they have achieved and enjoy their experience. If during the act of giving birth women are totally in tune with their bodies, a special hormonal flow is set up, and if nothing is allowed to interfere with it, many women actually feel an emotional high that can last for weeks after birth. To that extent, the way a woman is prepared for birth and how she experiences it, can in itself greatly influence how she feels in the postnatal period.

Differentiate between feeling depressed and being depressed

However, we need to be aware that a few women may develop clinical depression and that such women will feel unable to cope with looking after the baby or themselves, having lost interest in life and all motivation. There may have been a history of ambivalence towards the pregnancy, there may be emotional conflict in the couple's relationship. In caring for the child, early unhappy memories and experiences may surface causing pain and anguish which the mother may find crippling. There may be anger or resentment towards the mother's own mother, father, husband – or the child. These may cause nightmares, obsessive thoughts of killing herself, the husband or the baby. In such cases it is imperative that medical or psychiatric help is sought without delay. Clinical postnatal depression is treatable but needs proper professional attention.

Treatment may consist of medication or shock therapy or psychotherapy or a combination of any of these.

Antidepressant drugs should be distinguished from mere tranquillizers (like Valium). The latter do not bring about significant improvement and can lead to dependency.

One theory holds that clinical postnatal depression may be the result of a malfunction of the thyroid gland after birth and needs to be treated accordingly. Some women have derived dramatic benefits from hormone therapy. Other women found vitamin supplements of great help. Whatever drugs or vitamins are prescribed, great care has to be taken in the choice of medication as they can have varying effects on breastfeeding.

A caring and sympathetic doctor should be able to establish and determine what is of most help to the individual woman in this situation.

In summary, points to cover during antenatal teaching on this aspect:

○ distinguish between *feeling* or *being* depressed
○ weepiness is common and natural – list all possible reasons

○ helpful hints to cope with physiological changes (teas, cremes, herbal remedies, exercises, compresses etc.)

○ helpful hints to cope with emotional strains (beware visitors' intrusion in terms of time and unsolicited advice, give yourself time and space for love and attention)

○ destroy the media's myth of blissful motherhood

○ encourage flexibility, jettison all ideologies and take each day as it comes

○ enable couples to seek help, be it practical, medical or psychological.

Fear of handicap and death

Sometimes the issues of handicap and death come up by itself. If not you could bring it into a session when it seems suitable. One good lead in is the statement somebody makes in group and everybody readily agrees to: 'I don't mind what sex it is as long as it is healthy'. Why is ill health and death something that is so feared in our society?

To introduce or structure this theme you also can ask the participants: 'What would be the worst thing that could happen?' This can be answered either in the form of a 'flashlight', in pair work or in small groups. Then either in the whole group or in small groups explore the issues further using questions similar to the following:

– which type of handicap would be worst for us?
– what is it that frightens me?
– do I fear my inability to love a handicapped child?
– do I fear the rejection of neighbours, friends etc?
– do I fear the disappointment of my expectations?
– do I fear the change in my lifestyle?
– do I fear the strain on our marriage?
– how would we deal with it if it were reality?

Find examples of how acquaintances or others coped with having a handicapped child. How were their lives affected?

REFLECTIONS

The aims for working with this theme are:

1 Let yourself know what it is that you fear and to reflect how we would deal with it in reality (gradual elimination of fear through concretization).

2 Become more sensitive to the issues surrounding handicap and death and try to be able to be with somebody who is affected by handicap or death. One of the biggest problems of the persons affected is the isolation.

3 Attempt to integrate thoughts about death and handicap into your everyday life. They are part of life, and death in particular is what gives life its definition. They are not unnatural or evil and do not need to be excluded or denied.

Fear of death   Many people find it difficult to accept or to permit death or dying. Why should a dying child be forced to live? For whom is the child's life necessary? A reflection on why parents *need* the survival or health of their child? is important (see chapter on Preparation for parenthood),

Can we accept that perhaps people choose when they want to die?

Can we imagine and accept that a person just wanted to enjoy being carried by somebody else, to never outgrow its innocence? What a wonderful thought it is to be *inside* somebody else, to feel another person from within, in such closeness! Can we imagine a being that wants to go no further than that? That doesn't really want to live outside the womb (Stillbirth).

Can we imagine and understand that maybe somebody wanted to come to this world, wanted to love but then changed his or her mind and decided not to live after all? (Cot death) Can we grant to the child we love that it does not need to go further than it wants, that it can change its mind, that it does not have to live for us.

But trying to understand the baby is one thing. The bereaved parents need understanding too.

They might feel very guilty, blaming themselves for not having loved the unborn child, for not having wanted to be pregnant in the first few months, for having smoked too much during pregnancy etc. They might blame themselves for the choice of hospital or for having gone to the hospital too late. So many possible reasons. Parents want explanations why their child had to die and they often feel that they were the cause. 'If only I had . . .', or they need someone else to blame. The other feeling that the bereaved have to live with is that of rejection. 'The baby didn't like me, it didn't want to stay with me', 'I am not worthy to be a mother or father'.

To mention these likely reactions to prospective parents will help them to become sensitive to the issues of life and death.

Talking about this in class might enable them to contact a bereaved friend or neighbour instead of, as is so often the case, avoiding them.

The main problem for bereaved parents – besides coping with the loss – is the isolation. Very few friends or relatives can cope with the seemingly never ending stream of blame, anger and sadness, yet neither do they dare to invite them to parties or outings, because they find it inappropriate to suggest a light-hearted event. Another issue bereaved mothers often mention, is that nobody asks them about their labour. They have gone through it too and want to share their experience. Yet somehow, because there is no 'product' they are not included in the 'club of mothers'. Mothers who have lost their child may need to express their sadness and anger, but they also want to tell someone all the positive things they had experienced during labour. How well they coped with the strength of contractions, how pleasurable those early tingly sensations were, how loving the contact with their husband. It is important too to give bereaved parents the chance to talk of the time when the child was still alive, very much alive, kicking and responding. For it did live, even if only in the womb. In this context mention that should their baby be born dead, they should look at him, hold the baby, touch him/her and name him/her. And to take a photo too. Stillborn babies usually look very peaceful like a sleeping baby. If parents don't dare to look and hold and recognize they only have a false memory, and taunt themselves with gruesome images or else they deny the reality totally, don't grieve fully and perhaps never properly come to terms with the loss of their child. Sometimes participants (especially fathers) mention dreams about giving birth to strange monstrous beings. These dreams are not to be seen as premonition, but as a strengthening. Their psyche deals with the fear of the unknown.

We might like to believe that many deaths can be avoided — by optimal antenatal care, knowledge about the birth process, about necessary and avoidable interventions, and by choosing an optimal birthplace, midwife etc. But reality seems to prove that whilst a lot of complications can indeed be avoided, the life or death of a baby cannot be programmed. If a baby wants to live, it can survive the most adverse situations; if a baby needs to die, it will die, despite optimal precautions and surroundings. For example, by something totally unpredictable happening. We cannot plan life or death, but we can open ourselves for both experiences:
  – where do we come from?
  – what is the meaning of life?
  – what happens to us after we die?

These are essential questions in anybody's life. Even if we know the answer we could not give it to anyone else. But we can encourage people to address those questions to themselves, for everyone has an answer within.

Fear of handicap   Most people find it difficult to accept handicap, their own or that of others. But why is the lack of certain abilities described as 'being handicapped' whereas the absence of other abilities is considered 'normal'?
  – a child who cannot speak but can express him/herself exceptionally well with music or drawing is still called handicapped, yet a child who shows no musical or artistic talent at all and has no exceptional linguistic capacity either is still considered normal.
  – a person who can't walk but gets about in a wheelchair, enjoys his or her environment, the process of getting there and reaching the goal, is called handicapped, yet a person who can walk easily, but doesn't care where he or she is going, can't enjoy the environment, the process or the goal, is still considered normal.

Why is it more acceptable for most people to have a child of normal or above-average intelligence, who has problems in expressing him/herself emotionally, than to have a child with below-average intelligence but who can feel and express intensely feelings of gratitude, love and joy?

With this viewpoint you can encourage participants to look at the issue of handicap differently, to question their own 'normality' and superiority. Many 'handicapped' people develop superior abilities of one sort or another.

But you do not need to idealize; it is important to deal with the reality also:

- in addition to the original handicap of the child there is often a behavioural problem that results from the necessary institution-alization (of one sort or another) or the overprotection or rejection of his/her parents. It is often these behaviour problems that are more noticeable and disturbing than the original handicap.
- few marriages withstand the stress of living with a handicapped child. It is almost always the men who leave their wives because as mothers they are too absorbed with the child. A 'handicapped' child does alter the lifestyle of a family even more than a 'normal' child. It is usually the men who feel more threatened and challenged by their handicapped child. It is a challenge that most men avoid because other 'challenges' seem more important.

(This point is dynamite for every group discussion and touches issues beyond the subject of handicap).

In group discussions it often emerges that for women the fear of being left alone with a handicapped child is far greater than the fear of not being able to meet the needs of the child.

It is extremely difficult for parents to find playmates for their handicapped child. 'Normal' children of friends or neighbours are often scared of the unusual movements or noises the 'handicapped' child makes. It is very painful for parents to see how their handi-capped child gets rejected by other children even though their child longs for the contact and is full of love, openness and forgiveness.

Participants will find discussing these issues valuable and are most likely to remember what was talked about in class should they be confronted with handicap in reality. And a lot will have been achieved if only they encourage their own healthy children to play with a handicapped child in their neighbourhood. Assurance and guidance can also be offered regarding more or less serious or passing illnesses that newborn children can have (severe jaundice, pylonic stenosis etc). Perhaps using case histories (that you have gathered or partici-pants have contributed) you can talk about how affected parents dealt with the illness practically and emotionally.

An extended session — about fear of handicap, death and illness is of course only appropriate if there is energy for it in the group. When you introduce the session explain to the participants that you don't expect them to be confronted with death, handicap or severe illness, but that the purpose of the session is to help them deal with any fears they might have. But if there is really no desire for it, you can just mention the main points briefly and leave it at that.

Before you offer a session like this one, do look at the nature and intensity of your own fears so that these are not communicated unreflectively.

24　Sensitization of the partners to each other

Each labour is dependent on whether those involved are in unison with themselves and with each other. To be 'in unison' with oneself means to be *sensitive*, in touch with our mental, emotional and intuitive selves and their relatedness.

- If our mental level (intellect) is not connected with our emotions and our intuition we cannot act sensitively.
- If we are not aware of our emotions we are unable to use our intuition sensitively.
- If our intuition is distorted by our emotions (hate, inferiority etc.) we cannot use it sensitively.
- If we are not able to express our intuition it will remain implicit only.

There is the belief that mental knowledge gets in the way of true sensitivity. This is because sometimes we use our mental knowledge very insensitively by labelling, rationalizing, demoralizing, diminishing, distancing, undermining, overpowering others or ourselves. This happens when our emotions get in the way, when our unresolved anger, envy, insecurity, fear etc. hides behind knowledge; then we act insensitively. It is not the intellect but the desire to control that is opposed to sensitivity.

Sensitization has to do with attunement, with flow, with surrendering, with giving up control. This can be frightening to both men and women. Some men might not be able to relax in class because it is their very tense-ness, rationality and detachment that their wife needs, so that she can let go completely. For some women it is important to know that her partner does not 'lose his head'. Only in the safety of that knowledge can they relax into their bodies.

REFLECTIONS　1 Can you allow yourself both to be in touch with your bodies simultaneously, to surrender to each other, to stop being in control? or does it feel safer and right for you if only one at a time surrenders and the other one stays in control?

Even if partners choose the latter for themselves — i.e. that the woman should 'learn to surrender' for birth, whereas the man wants to remain in control — we can still invite the man to explore and experiment with surrendering. To be able to let go completely in class does not mean that the man will want to do that at birth too.

Another belief is that the 'regression', that women can enter at birth (which enables the flow of tranquillizing hormones), can only happen if there is no cerebral functioning required. Experience shows however that in fact regression is often paired with mental clarity in labouring women. Regression is wrongly paired with non-thinking! Gradually we grant newborn children more intellectual abilities than were admitted before. But when it comes to regression in labouring women, suddenly again we deny them their thinking abilities. Feelings of fear, mistrust, anger etc., rather than thinking, interfere with this regression. In order for feelings not to interfere these sensitization exercises come in useful.

2 What does it mean to you to sensitize partners to each other?

3 What would you call a sensitive partner?
How much sensitivity do you expect and get from your partner?
What does sensitivity mean to you personally?
Which of the following types of sensitivity are important to you and in which order?

- ○ Your partner senses what you feel and want
- ○ Your partner is able to give you what you need at the right time
- ○ The touch of your partner has a certain quality
- ○ Your partner is sensitive towards his own needs
- ○ . . . .(what would be your 'definition'?).

4 Which types of sensitivity would you expect from the couples in your classes and which would you like to show?

It is important that our own expectation and experience with our own partner does not get transferred to the couples in class. Every relationship has its own pattern and what might seem coarse and insensitive to one, could be the optimum for another.

Sometimes the antenatal teacher tries to sensitize the couples whilst remaining, herself, rather insensitive to the group process and to the real needs of the individuals. Again, no amount of knowledge or the application of perfected techniques can create sensitivity. We cannot make people sensitive. We can only be sensitive. It is our *own* sensitivity that sensitizes the couples, not the sensitization exercises that we might use.

You do not have to use any of the following exercises. It all depends on *how* you introduce and evaluate anything you do. Just as you can use the teaching of a breathing or massage technique *as a* sensitization exercise so any of the following exercises can easily be reduced to the presentation of another *technique*.

EXERCISE

QUESTIONNAIRE

Questionnaire: How do you expect your partner to react at birth?

The questionnaire should contain at least six different situations so that there are opportunities for expressing divergent points of view. Ask all the participants to underline what they think they or their partners would do in that situation.

Suggest partners sit back to back while making their notes. Not only does this avoid the premature comparing of notes, but it enhances the feelings of both individuality and togetherness. Afterwards couples can face each other and compare notes and explain why they expected a certain reaction from themselves or their partners and what it would mean to them if this expectation was not fulfilled.

Examples:

You are in labour. You arrive at hospital. The midwife tells the husband to go to the waiting room until he is called, saying: 'Surely you don't want to be around while your wife is getting an enema'.
He goes to the waiting room/You go to the waiting room
○ Definitely   ○ Perhaps   ○ Definitely not

You are in first stage of labour walking round in the delivery room. Hugging and rocking gently with each contraction. Both you and your partner feel OK with it. The midwife says: 'Well Mrs . . . . . . you better lie down now, all that walking about is too exhausting'.

She lies down/You lie down
○ Definitely   ○ Perhaps   ○ Definitely not

EXERCISE

BACK TO BACK

Pair exercise.

Duration: 5–7 min.

Sit on the floor, back to back, leaning against each other.

Breathe through and out.

Move your back a bit to be comfortable, change your position until you feel you're sitting really well.

Relax your head and neck and shoulders.

Breathe in and out.

Now become aware of your back and your partner's back.

Are you more supporting or more supported?

Which of you is more supporting or more supported?

Be aware of little nuances.

Who is leaning more?

You can always change your position a bit.

Slowly, begin to find a movement together, swinging gently with your upper body into various directions, stronger or more lightly.

Feel what is more, what is less, pleasant.

Feel which of you is more guiding, which more guided?

Let yourselves know how you feel about this.

Would you like a more intense movement but don't dare take the initiative?

Would you like a gentler movement but don't dare resist your partner?

Continue moving with each other.

Explore different patterns, different rhythms.

Experiment a bit together, create new patterns.

Be aware of your contact and of your feelings with the movement.

Who is guiding? Who is following?

Experiment a bit more together.

What do you find pleasant? What do you find unpleasant?

And then, slowly allow the movement to come to rest.

And just sit, leaning against each other's back.

Become aware again of how your contact feels.

Then breathe deeply and 'peel' yourself from your partner's back.

Duration: 3–5 min.

Now face each other and share what you experienced. Tell your partner what you liked and what you did not like about your own and about his behaviour. Tell him/her what you wished you or he/she had done.

Conclude with a group discussion or 'Flashlight': what did everybody experience? Possibly bring in reflections, questions yourself, if there is interest.

Questions after the exercise
- is resistance not also control? (partner can't do what he/she wants to)
- is surrendering not also control? (only then can the activity flow, happen)
- do I need the resistance of the partner to remain active?
- will his or her surrender make me inactive?
- is there a clear role division in the relationship?
- does every partner take his/her turn in leading?
- do I like my own behaviour?
- do I like the behaviour of my partner?
- what would I like to change?
- what would I like him/her to change?
- how do I imagine our relationship pattern during labour?
- how would I like to be/to behave?
- how would I like him/her to be/to behave?

There are different ways of supporting and each partner has to find out for him/herself what suits him/her and also the relationship best.

○ I can support with strain, being active
○ I can support through letting go completely myself, being passive.

Repeat the pair exercise guiding the couples with similar words again, to give them a chance to try out and explore new patterns with each other.

This could then be followed by a talk about what the partners expect from each other during birth (control, support, activity, passivity etc.) and what sort of behaviour they expect from themselves.

Another way to explore the theme of control and surrender within the pair relationship is the following variation.

EXERCISE

DANCE WITH FINGERTIPS

Couple (A and B) stand opposite each other, about armslength apart.

Palms of hands touching at shoulder height. Both step back an inch, so that only the fingertips remain in contact.

Either B only or both close their eyes.

A begin to make movements with your hands (making sure not to lose B's fingertips right at the beginning).
A become increasingly daring, moving your arms, forward, backward, sideways, up, down, in bigger or smaller circles, figure of eight, any shape and rhythm that you can think of.

B follow the movement so that both your fingertips always stay in touch.

Without verbal exchange change over after 2–3 min.

Now B divert the movements and A try to follow the movement.

Become aware of how you feel in guiding and being guided.

How trusting or how confident are you in your respective roles?

In the ensuing discussion you can ask:
- did you enjoy the movements?
- which 'dance' did you enjoy more, the one that you guided or the one that you were guided in?
- would you have liked to make other movements, but found your partner prevented you from trying them out?
- did you find it easy to follow the guidance?
- did you expect a different 'dance'?
- could you accept that the 'dance' you did experience, was different but therefore not necessarily bad?
- did you feel you inwardly criticized your partner for being different and/or not living up to your expectations?
- did you resist your partner's movements even though you enjoyed them?
- do you see parallels in your everyday relationship?

EXERCISE

TRUST EXERCISE IN A CIRCLE

Create two circles, one outer and an inner one. Everyone sit on the floor facing the centre. The partner of each person in the inner circle sit behind your partner in the outer circle.

Those in the inner circle close their eyes and relax.

The partner in the outer circle put your hands on the back of the person in front of you.

Touch, stroke, massage.

Make contact through touch.

Transmit trust through touch.

Eventually feel more daring.

(Set in motion the back of the person in front of you)

Swing it rhythmically.

Gather it backwards into your own lap.

The person in the inner circle: try to surrender completely.

Try to trust and enjoy the caress and stimulation you receive.

Now those in the outer circle steady the back of your partners again in an upright position and gradually remove your hands.

Change over

Share the experience in the pair relationship.

Possibly follow up with a 'flashlight' or group discussion.

EXERCISE

TUCKING UP AND BEING TUCKED UP

A sits somewhere on the floor, eyes closed, relaxing.

B prepares a bed for A just behind or next to him or her, with cushions, blanket etc.

A allows B to be placed on that 'bed' and to be tucked up.

A does absolutely nothing: neither supports him or herself nor moves any part of his or her body into a more comfortable position, nor gives any sort of sign of what feels right or not right.

B moves A's body into a side, front, or back position with cushions under the head, arms, legs or anywhere he or she thinks they are wanted.

B moves the limbs and head of A until B feels that he or she found the optimal position for A to fall asleep in.

A accepts being moved about, neither helping nor resisting any change of position.

A lets him- or her*self* know what this position feels like, what he or she would want changed, but does not say so yet!

B having done his or her best, now asks for feedback and suggestions.

A can *now* request as much as he or she likes ('Can you move my head slightly to the right . . . I'd like to lie on my back . . . .Could you place my legs a bit further apart, no not quite as far as that . . .. No I'd rather lie curled up . . .' etc.) again doing nothing to assist the adjustments.

B allows him, or herself to feel his or her reactions to those requests (irritability, guilt for not having done it better in the first place, anger about the other person's demands etc.) but does not say so yet.

A experiences his or her feelings in making requests. (Shyness at having to . . . pleasure in being allowed to . . .) without talking about it.

A thanks B when finally the perfect tucking up position is achieved.

The partners exchange their experiences with one another.

Not to be able to say anything in the earlier stages of the exercise intensifies the awareness of one's emotions.

Follow up with a 'flashlight' or group discussion on the issues of 'trust', 'asking for something', 'responding' or whatever became important for the participants.

To further the reflection introduce questions like:
- how easy was it for you to know whether your partner felt good in the position you chose for him or her?
- did you enjoy having the power to give?
- did you enjoy tuning in to your partner?
- did you allow your partner to bodily manipulate you?
- could you accept somebody else doing something for you?

EXERCISE

TO TRUST AND TO DARE

This is quite a delicate and important pair exercise.
Use a volunteer to demonstrate.

A lies relaxed on his or her back, possibly with a cushion or wedge under back and head to avoid heartburn in late pregnancy.

B lifts, stretches and manipulates the limbs and head of A. You can either explain in detail what you are doing as you are demonstrating the exercise or you can give them very detailed instructions as they are doing it.

Instructions to A

Just lie completely relaxed.

Give yourself time to get calm and relaxed.

Breathe out.

Let go of any tension with your outbreath.

Let yourself know inside how ready you are for the manipulations that are about to happen to your body.

Breathe deeply; breathe out.

Become aware of a part in you that is open and trusting.

Let go completely of any holding back.

Do nothing for the next 10 min.

Allow your partner to help you soften and open physically.

Just allow this openness to happen.

Instructions to B

Find a space for yourself next to the right foot of your partner. Try kneeling or sitting however you are most comfortable. Make sure you are not sitting too close.

Breathe deeply; breathe out.

Observe whether you are really comfortable and centred in your position.

Allow yourself to be relaxed.

Now observe the breathing of your partner; tune in.

With the next outbreath of your partner lift his or her leg, supporting the hollow of the knee with your right hand and the heel with your left hand.

Lift the leg as high as you are comfortable with, leaning backwards with your own body, so that you exert a slight pull, not with the strength of your arm muscles, but effortlessly by leaning back a little bit, gently and gradually move the leg about a bit as you pull it gently with your own body weight. Up and down, sideways, in a circling motion, in larger and smaller circles. Don't exaggerate, only as much as feels comfortable for yourself.

Don't force anything; stay in touch with how much your partner is prepared to let go.

Don't pull with your arms but just continuously lean back, so that you never push the leg towards the pelvic frame.

Gradually, lower the leg again with gentle swinging motion and bring it to rest on the ground outstretched.

Now with each of your partner's outbreaths stroke the whole leg from the pelvis to beyond the toes, in one long sweeping motion, and again, firmly or very softly as it feels right to you.

Repeat with the left leg. Make sure you are sitting comfortably, not too close to the left leg of your partner.

Now sit next to the left arm, observe how comfortable you are.

Focus on your breathing.

With the next outbreath of your partner gently lift the arm holding the left hand with your right hand. As soon as the elbow lifts off the ground support it with your left hand.

Now gently pull the whole arm towards you again, by leaning back.

Only exert as much pull as you need to loosen the joint, but without pulling the upper body towards you.

Move the arm with gentle pulling motion upwards, sideways, in larger and smaller circles. With a slight swinging motion lower the arm gently, placing it outstretched on the ground.

Stroke the arm rhythmically a few times from the shoulder to beyond the fingertips. As the arm is resting on the ground take just the hand in your left hand and with your right hand gently pull each individual finger in a very slight turning motion. Don't exert strength, just gently stretch each finger of the left hand making sure you don't push the arm back towards the shoulder as you do so.

Repeat with the right arm and hand of your partner.

Make sure that you are sitting comfortably and are relaxed.

Tune in to your breathing and the breathing of your partner.

Find a good space just behind your partner's head, kneeling or sitting crosslegged, which ever is more comfortable.

Observe your own position and breathing. Become centred and relaxed yourself.

Now gently place your left hand under your partner's neck, stroking outwards as you remove your hand again. Alternate this a few times, with your right and left hand moving any hair out of the neck area as you stroke outwards.

Gently roll the head sideways, still on the ground. Place both hands supporting each other under your partner's neck and lift the head very gradually and gently, while exerting a very slight pull.

Move the head gently up and down and sideways, in very slow motion and without ever letting the weight of the head push into the neck. You hold the whole weight in your hands (see illustration)

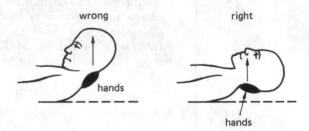

With a slight swinging motion lower the head again and place it, neck slightly stretched, on the ground.

Now with each outbreath of your partner stroke your partner a few times from the neck up the back of the head to beyond the end of the hair.

Quiet Reflection

Both of you rest for a few minutes and become aware of the effects of this exercise inside you.

– how do you feel as A: could you let go, and give yourself over
to your partner?
– did you feel inner resistance? – when?
– with which parts of your body did you find it most difficult to
open and let go?
– with which parts of your body was it easy for you?
– how much trust did you feel in your partner?
– at the beginning of the exercise? – during? – and now?
– how do you feel as B: how much did you dare to bring out of
your partner? – do you feel it was too much, too little or just
right?
– with which parts of your partner's body did you find it most
difficult?
– with which body parts was it easy for you?
– how much confidence did you feel? – at the beginning of the
exercise? – during? – and now?

Verbal Reflection
(5 min)

In this exchange within the pair relationship it can be useful to
encourage a special form of feedback using only 'I' statements.

Instead of:	use
'You did that well'	'I felt good'
'You pulled my arms too much'	'I couldn't let my arms go'
'Your legs were tense'	'I had difficulties with your legs'
	etc.

Then change over: A is B, and B is A
Duration of exercise including reflection and following flashlight
30–40 min.

TO BE MORE OPEN AND HONEST IN THE SEXUAL RELATIONSHIP

EXERCISE

Men's and women's group:
– what do I wish for sexually from my partner?

In their respective groups men and women collect and note down
their wishes. After 10–15 min. (depending on how intensively the
group work develops) the groups sit facing each other. A speaker
from each reads aloud the collected wishes to the other group
without mentioning names (though they can differentiate): 'All of
us would like . . .' 'Some of us wish for . . .' 'One of us wishes . . .'

This exercise is great for stimulating further thoughts, and talk on
the way home. Over and over again when doing this exercise in

classes, it becomes obvious that men are able to formulate their wishes quite concretely ('She should stroke my arms'; 'She shouldn't hold me so tight during orgasm'; 'She should bite my back.' . . . etc.); whereas women express more vague wishes: asking for more tenderness, more hugging and kissing, longer foreplay etc. It is interesting that even when this exercise is done with a class of women only divided into two groups, one of the groups playing the role of men, even those 'men' are able to express their wishes more explicitly.

If there is time and interest suggest that each group works for another 10 minutes in order to fantasize and concretize what 'More tenderness . . .' 'Longer foreplay', etc means. (To kiss the inside of my elbow' . . . To stroke her earlobes' . . . etc.) What often happens is that the women collect wishes for what *he* should *not do* ('Not to pull my hair'; 'Not to breathe into my ears'; 'Not to push my head into the pillow etc.) rather than what '*I* would *like* him to *do*'. Although these 'negative' points are equally valid (and often women have made a secret of their dislikes for years) it is a point which reinforces the comment above; that even when they do decide to express themselves directly, women will still tend to hide behind the negative (not do) rather than stick their necks out and ask for what they really want. Of course, this behaviour (which *is* socially conditioned — as girls women are taught to be quiet and demure and passive) extend way outside the field of sexual relationships, into all aspects of everyday living. With some reflection, encouragement and roleplay women can be encouraged to become more assertive, and more able to ask for what they want regardless (accepting) of the consequences. It is important that this too gets expressed. Many women might have kept their dislikes secret for many years. Usually I sit together with the women's group in that phase and encourage them to become really explicit about what they would like their partner to know (for example: to only rub and stroke the skin folds around the clitoris, the clitoris itself gets easily sore, when touched directly. Men mostly just know that the clitoris is the 'button' for turn on but don't know how to trigger it).

If, as it sometimes happens, the men's groups also formulates rather vague wishes in the first phase of the exercise, (she should be more active – she should dress more attractively etc.), in which case both groups should concretize their own wishes in the second phase.

EXERCISE

SILENT REFLECTION

Make a list, written as explicitly as possible (partners sitting back to back again) of all your wishes: those you often said or never expressed, those that are fulfilled or that remain unfulfilled so far . . . you will not have to show this list to anybody.

I would like you to . . .   I don't like it, if you . . .

. . .   . . .

. . .   . . .

Allow 10 min. to complete the list. Then looking at your list consider the following:
  – which wishes have I never expressed, and yet are fulfilled? (sometimes; often; always)
  – which wishes have I never expressed and which are never fulfilled?
  – how important are these wishes to me?
  – which wishes have I expressed and yet are still not fulfilled? Did I express them once/more than once/often?

Turn to your partner and explore what stops you from expressing your wishes.

You can use the 'rosary' method ('I fear, that . . .) or the questioning method (Why can't you tell me your wishes?)

As a next step, and more effectively done as homework, suggest to the couples to use the rosary or questioning method at home to explore what it is they wish for from each other.

EXERCISE

TO OBSERVE AND TO NAME FEELINGS

Duration: 15 min.

This pair exercise helps the couple not only to become more aware of each other but is a good preparation for understanding their baby later on. The baby can't express itself clearly and verify its feelings in words.

The couple just sit opposite each other silently for a few minutes looking at each other, observing any trace of expression in each other's face.

After a few minutes they describe to each other what they perceive.

Example

  I could see one part of you that is tired, a bit restless, annoyed maybe, another part of you feels satisfied and quite pleased. Somewhere in you is sadness about something . . ..

When they have both voiced their observations each can then verify or amend the statements.

In the ensuing group discussion it is valuable to point out how easy it is to project our own feeling onto others, or to see only what we want to see.

You and the group might want to repeat the exercise, just to check whether participants are able to see in their partners what the partners say they feel. It is a challenge too actually to show what one is feeling. Most of us are so 'clever' in hiding our feelings and yet end up surprised or annoyed that nobody 'sees'.

EXERCISE

TO COMMUNICATE SILENTLY

Through our eyes and with our facial expression we can tell our partner anything we want him or her to know. We can also get in contact with our own feelings and inner being by having been given space and silence to do so.

The task is to remain in eye contact for 6 min. The partners sit opposite each other, just looking at each other.

Min 1 + 2: A is sending his/her feelings about him/herself, about B, about anything that is important at the moment. B is the receiver. Just looking and observing A's face and eyes openly and intently.

Min. 3 + 4: the roles are reversed. B is sending A is receiving.

Min 5 + 6: A and B communicate with their eyes simultaneously, both sending and receiving.

Neither partner interferes in any way by speaking or gesturing or avoid being in real contact with each other by chatting theorising or explaining the feelings away. Often when we speak we betray with our words our true intentions, we fool ourselves and our partners, often, when we hug each other, we avoid actually 'taking the other in'. It is often easier to hug somebody, looking over their shoulders, instead of looking into their eyes.

Verbal communication or physical closeness is important, but a real open and honest communication seems to happen best via the eyes (Is).

EXERCISE

TO OPEN AND TO ACCEPT HELP

In this pair exercise you can explore four different ways of helping the partner to open up, to loosen up physically. Both the helper and the helped can reflect upon which type of 'help' suits each best.

Ask yourselves:
  – when do you feel most or least resistance?
  – which type of help is experienced as most or least effective
    — both from the 'helper' and 'helped' point of view.

1. Pressure

A sits in butterfly position (on the floor, soles of feet touching) allowing knees to fall apart as far as possible, and leans back onto her hands.
B sits opposite and places ankles on top of A's knees, leaves the weight of his legs resting there for one minute.

Reflect on the pain you are causing and experiencing, how effective the pressure is or might be in allowing A to open towards or despite the pain. Do you believe that the greater the pain, the greater the effect?
Change places.

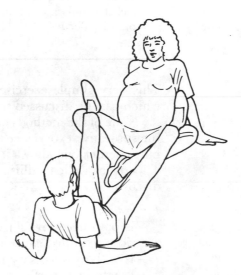

2. Action

A see above.
B kneels in front of A enclosing A's feet between his/her knees (to prevent them from slipping off). B places one hand under each knee of A, lifts the knees up (A's feet remain on the ground), bobs them up and down gently and lets them fall apart, lifts them again, loosens through bobbing and lets them fall again . . . a few times.

Reflect on how effective you experience this way of helping to be. Is the activity irritating, preventing real letting go? Does the opening happen with each surprise 'fall'? Do both believe that the greater the activity, the greater the effect?
Change places.

3. Warmth

A see above.
B kneels in front of A and places his/her hands just left and right of the pubic bone on the inside of A's thighs. Leans gently forward with the weight of his/her body

Reflect on how effective you experience the warmth and gentle pressure. Does it feel too 'close' and prevent A from really opening up? Do you both believe that the greater the intimacy and warmth, the greater the effect?
Change places.

4. Pressure, action and warmth

A see above.
B kneels in front of A and massages with each outbreath of A, the inside of A's thighs from the pubic bone to beyond the knees gradually increasing the pressure towards the knee, several times.

Reflect on how effective you experience this massage. Do you feel that only a combination of warmth, intimacy, pressure and pain is effective?

This very simple exercise brings into the open many of our beliefs which can be discussed in the large group.

None of the methods of help is objectively better than another: it is the subjective experience that counts. It is not the method that works, but whether one allows it to work.

You can elicit, affirm and question the beliefs that participants discovered.

For example
    – is pain necessary for change to come about?
    – does pain just cause tension and prevent progress?
    – is activity necessary for change to come about?
    – is activity superfluous and irritating and preventing real progress?
    – do I need help? Can I change on my own?
    – can I change — even when somebody is around expecting progress?
    – do I need a partner who is just there, calm and uninterfering?
    – do I need a partner, who is active and demanding?

None of these beliefs is objectively better than the other. Beliefs can change. Believing one thing today doesn't mean we have to stick to it. We have to remain aware and observe our reality. If we are not happy with the results that our beliefs create, it's time to change them.

25 Practising self-assertiveness

As with most aspects of our life we can only assert ourselves if we know what we want. If we ourselves are not sure about something, be it having a home delivery or not or remaining upright in labour, how can we assert ourselves?

As long as we are not sure of what we want we waste energy in an argument that is bound to end unsatisfactorily. If we really know what we want it is quite easy to be assertive. Quite often people think they have to learn certain rules of communication in order to assert themselves better, whereas in fact what they need is an awareness of their needs and desires.

Once we know what we want there are different approaches to letting others know.

To request or deny

Depending on our individual backgrounds we tend to slip into certain patterns of communication if we have to request or deny something. We can become:
- the dependent child
- the defiant child
- the bossy child
- the mature adult

EXAMPLE

The midwife asks the labouring woman to lie down ('You're only exhausting yourself, dear'). The woman's different reactions could be:
- to lie down – because she feels exhausted
- to lie down – because she doesn't dare object
- to ask 'Couldn't I remain standing,' because she's not sure want she wants.

Assuming she is sure she wants to remain standing, she can say:
  – 'Please let me stand just for a little while longer'.
  (The dependent child goes down well with many midwives. She may treat you like a child from now on, either with compliance or by ordering you about).
    – 'but I want to remain standing!' (defiant child, usually arouses stubbornness on part of the midwife too, which can lead to arguments. She often ends up being the loser, either because the midwife wins or because she 'wins' but ends up working with a midwife who lets her feel her rejection).
    – 'I don't care what you say, I remain in the position I want'. (bossy child, will provoke a response according to the personality structure of the midwife. She might respect you for your strength and become submissive, or she might get all her own bossyness out, or she might end up ignoring you most of the time, as you know better anyway).
    – 'I understand your concern but I want to remain standing for the time being. I will take care not to exhaust myself'. (adult self which has most chance of being accepted and respected).

But what happens, if the midwife should insist on your lying down, despite your adult response? That's where the rules of assertive communication become important:

1 Acknowledge that you heard what she said ('mirror')
2 Repeat simply what you want ('broken record')

Because:
If you were just to say 'I'd rather stay standing' the midwife will feel the need to repeat her reasoning assuming you didn't understand her concern: 'But you will exhaust yourself if you don't lie down'. On the other hand, if you were to say 'I'm not exhausted' she might look for signs of proof for her argument, 'But I can see you are tired/shivering/pale' etc. or go on to find the next reason 'It's better for your baby' etc. Whereas if you were to say 'I read that an upright position is better in labour' or try to give any other reason for *why* you are standing up you are just inviting an argument. All you need to say and to be clear about is *what you want*.

EXAMPLE OF DIALOGUE

Midwife: You'd better lie down now, Mrs X
Woman: Thank's, I want to remain standing
Midwife: It is better for you if you lie down now
Woman: It might be better for some women, but I know I feel better if I remain standing
Midwife: It is routine in this clinic, once you are here, you lie down.

Woman: Most women might lie down routinely but I want to
          remain standing.
Midwife: You will get totally exhausted.
Woman: I understand your concern that it could be
          exhausting but I feel better in this position and I
          want to remain standing up.

Eventually the midwife runs out of arguments and lets you remain in
your chosen position or she'll call the doctor and you might have to
re-run the communication until the doctor runs out of arguments.

Unfortunately though, the obstetric staff — if they want to remain
in power rather than listen to the individual woman's needs — have
other means to get you to lie down. 'Now you have to lie down,
because I need to do an internal examination/listen to the baby's
heart'. But a skilled and adaptable midwife can do both while you
remain upright, so this isn't a real argument. But for the sake of peace
and because she might have never examined a woman in an upright
position and feel genuinely insecure about it (yet, there always has to
be a first time) you can agree to lie down. 'For a few minutes, I do
want to get up again as soon as the examination is over'. And in a
normal labour progress there is no reason why you shouldn't.
However, if you choose to lie down, you might well find it comfortable
and be happy to remain lying for a while or for good, which is fine.
Don't feel you lose face, follow you body's signals at any time. If you
feel genuinely uncomfortable, get up again. Some woman are able to
'hold back' their labour progress by remaining upright. As soon as
they lie down a certain 'giving in' happens and contractions get
spontaneously stronger, more effective and more painful. So be aware
of whether you want to get up to avoid painfully effective contractions — a choice that doesn't serve you well in the long run of
labour — or whether you want to get up, becaue you know you will
just get all tense and upset while lying down and will slow labour that
way. The latter is a reason for getting up again and finding a position
where you can let go. In the reality of obstetric care unfortunately yet
another argument can be brought in at that point.

The midwife or doctor can pretend the baby isn't well, so they
need to listen to its heartbeat continuously, which means continuous
monitoring, which might require your lying down.

Now this could be true or it could just be a power game. If their
objection is genuinely the need for monitoring the baby and the
contractions, and they don't really mind whether you are upright or
lying down, you could be monitored in an upright position, if you
insist.

They just need to attach the electronic equipment to you, while
lying down and then help you into an upright position on, or next to
the bed, without getting the cables tangled up.

Everything can be solved if you know what you want and there is a
willingness to cooperate from the obstetric staff. You can apply the
above rules of communication, to assert yourself in requesting the
hospital of your choice or a home birth, or anything else in fact.

EXAMPLE

Doctor:	Now Mrs X, I have booked you into Hospital A
Woman:	I have looked at some hospitals, and I would like to be booked into Hospital B
Doctor:	But all the women of this area go into Hospital A
Woman:	I know most women go into hospital A but I would like to go to Hospital B
Doctor:	It is very complicated to get you booked into a hospital outside this area.
Woman:	I know it is difficult but not impossible and I do want to go to Hospital B
Doctor:	Well I don't know whether I am able to do this, I will try/could you make your own arrangements?

To request and deny

Assertiveness will only benefit you if you have awareness. Awareness about what you want. Awareness about your choices and options. Awareness about what's going on in reality.

To respond to criticism

It is difficult for most of us to deal with criticism. We might accept it too readily. It might hurt, but not help us. It might trigger our anger, rejection, refusal to listen etc. By and large, we tend to interpret it negatively rather than constructively. We all have our different defence mechanism that prevents us from learning and changing and entering an open communication.

REFLECTION

Write down about 5 phrases of criticism that you hear regularly from friends, partner, colleagues, parents, etc. or some phrases that you heard once, yet haven't forgotten. Now look at that list of criticisms and check through them:
  – which of them are true?
  – which of them are not true?

Once you have divided them into those two groups check through again:
  – which of them really hurt (whether or not they are true)?

Then let yourself know:
  – what do you feel about it?

Pick out some sentences that are important to you and write a response stating
  – whether or not it is true

– whether it hurts you
– what you feel about it

EXAMPLE

'You have no sense of humour'
Yes, that is true. I know that I am far too serious most of the
time and I would like myself to be more humorous.

'You are getting fatter every day'
I know it is true, I am overweight. I don't like it myself, but it
does hurt me very much if you say it to me like that.

Responding to criticism in such a way — i.e. by evaluating what is
said without defence — is disarming, avoids unnecessary arguments,
and makes you feel better about yourself. You are asserting yourself.
   Find some responses to the following criticisms you could be
confronted with in antenatal care or labour.

'Ooh you don't look very big. You should eat more, exercise less'
'You are putting your baby at risk with your unreasonable
demands.'
'Now you have shifted position again, I told you to lie still
otherwise the monitor won't work.'

There are participants in each class who have been confronted by
criticisms that they would like to share and to explore a good response
for it.
   You can use little roleplays to practise assertive responses.

26 Preparation for parenthood

It is not always easy to get pregnant couples interested in the reality of parenthood. Their thoughts and feelings seem all bound with the theme of birth. It is almost as though they can't — or daren't (maybe there's subconscious superstition here) see beyond the birth. Nevertheless it is important to encourage the pregnant couples to focus on the time beyond birth, on parenthood and the reality of child care.

The following examples of how to introduce or structure the session on preparation for parenthood do not aim to create a group consensus on what parenting should be like (e.g., babies should get used to a regular sleeping pattern; babies should be carried around as much as possible etc.) but rather encourage the participants to communicate about such issues. In the safe environment of the class participants can experiment with solving conflict situations. They can explore how they want to deal with the questions of child rearing. The aim of this session is also that neither of them is left alone, with having to find the solutions themselves. But to experience the fun, creativity and challenge of parenting together. If a couple decides that one of them will take on the role of the decisionmaker, then this should be a conscious decision for both partners.

Reflect on the exercises you introduce, whether you tend to impress 'right' or 'wrong' ways of parenting. There are no right answers that are of value to everybody.

Or are there?

Check out your own beliefs.

Make a list of right answers that contain validity for 'mankind' in your eyes.

Be aware of the values that you are passing on.

EXERCISE

QUESTIONNAIRE ON PARENTING

Develop your own questionnaire that suits the constellation of your classes (whether you teach single mothers, couples or women who come without their partners) and the problem situations they are likely to encounter.

In a couples class, ask the couples to sit back to back to one another to enhance their feeling of separateness and togetherness while they fill in the questionnaire. Afterwards, they can face each other and choose one issue where their points of view are opposed. They can now explain to one another why they chose their particular answer and look jointly for a solution that is satisfying for all three of them, taking the possible needs of the baby into account as well.

In a class solely of women you can ask two women to sit together to compare their answer and discuss one of the issues where their opinions differ. Sometimes it is only after expressing one's decision or hearing another point of view that one is able to become aware of what one's individual standpoint really is.

In the ensuing group discussion you can reflect on how decisionmaking comes about and which possible solutions exist for individual parents.

Each question in the questionnaire contains certain implicit values that are important to be aware of. For example in Questionnaire B the first question implies that the couple will breastfeed, the second question implies that the mother is with the baby most of the time, the third question implies that bringing the baby into one's bed could be a solution, the fourth question implies the father is practically involved in parenting.

This questionnaire was developed as it fitted the values of most of the participants, but it is nevertheless important to make this implication explicit so that the participants have a chance to reflect on their *own* values. They do not have to conform.

EXERCISE

EXAMPLES FOR A QUESTIONNAIRE: A

1 Your baby is one week old. It is afternoon. You have just settled your baby after a feed. She started crying within seconds. She seems to cry as soon as you put her down and stops as soon as you pick her up again. What will you do?

Pick up your baby
○ definitely/○ probably/○ maybe

Let your baby cry
○ maybe/○ probably/○ definitely

What other solution could you envisage . . .?

2 Your baby is six weeks old. You have taken your baby for daily walks in the fresh air so far. Now it has got rather chilly, what will you do?

Stay at home with your baby
○ definitely/○ probably/○ maybe

Continue to take baby outdoors
○ maybe/○ probably/○ definitely

What other solution could you envisage . . .?

3 Your baby is nine weeks old. It is night time. Your baby usually wakes every three to four hours to breastfeed. You wake up as your breasts overflow. It is 5 hours since the last feed and the baby still sleeps. What will you do?

Wake your baby
○ definitely/○ probably/○ maybe

Let your baby sleep
○ maybe/○ probably/○ definitely

What other solution could you envisage (hand express the milk?) . . .?

4 At home your baby is peaceful and hardly ever cries. But every time you visit somebody, your baby screams for most of the time. This happened to you three times in a row. What will you do?

Stay home for the near future
○ definitely/○ probably/○ maybe

Continue to visit friends
○ maybe/○ probably/○ definitely

What other solution could you envisage . . .?

5 Most of your friends are smokers. Since the birth of the baby you don't like smoking in your home. What will you do?

Suffer silently
○ definitely/○ probably/○ maybe

Ask friends not to smoke in your home
○ maybe/○ probably/○ definitely

What other solution could you envisage . . .?

EXERCISE

EXAMPLES FOR A QUESTIONNAIRE: B

1 Your wife is breastfeeding on demand. Your mother, who fed you and your siblings in a 4-hour routine, is on a visit. When your wife is about to breastfeed your baby again after 2 hours, your mother is appalled and interferes. What will you do?

Support your wife's action
○ definitely/○ probably/○ maybe

Support your mother's reaction
○ maybe/○ probably/○ definitely

What other solution could you envisage . . .?

2 Your wife goes out on her own once a week. During that time you attend to the baby. Each time the baby cries for about 15 minutes before it accepts a bottle from you (expressed milk or formula) What will you do?

Ask your wife not to go out until baby is older
○ definitely/○ probably/○ maybe

Don't tell your wife about it so that she enjoys her time out
○ maybe/○ probably/○ definitely

What other solutions could you envisage . . .?

3 Your wife brings your baby into bed when it wakes at night. When you mention this to colleagues they react strongly and tell you, that this would spoil your baby and she would never want to sleep on her own. What will you do?

You are glad that they confirm your opinion and go home reinforced
○ definitely/○ probably/○ maybe

You contradict them
○ maybe/○ probably/○ definitely

What other solution could you envisage . . .?

4 You enjoy bathing and dressing your baby. Unfortunately each time you do so your wife criticizes you for something or other, you forgot to wipe baby's ears, you didn't dress her warmly enough, the nappies are put on too loosely . . .. What will you do?

Feel angry and stop bathing and dressing your baby
○ definitely/○ probably/○ maybe

Not feel attacked and go on enjoying the bathing and dressing
○ maybe/○ probably/○ definitely

What other solutions could you envisage . . .?

This questionnaire should also be filled in by the women, visualizing how their partner might react and then comparing their expectations.

EXERCISE

SITUATIONAL REFLECTIONS

Any one of the questionnaire type questions can be asked to introduce a particular theme (breastfeeding, needs of parents versus needs of child, joint parenting, etc.).

Example

It is 3am. You fed your baby half an hour ago. You know it's reasonably dry and not too warm or cold. Now it begins to whimper in its cot. What would you do?

The descriptions of such concrete situations easily trigger lively discussion. The disadvantage of this type of exercise is the tendency to search for a solution that is right for everyone. The problem of any large group work is to invite conformity. On the other hand the advantage is that you can collect a multitude of views (in this example, why a baby might cry) and solutions. It depends on how you handle the discussions. After introducing one example and its discussion you can invite the participants to share or invent their own examples of possible problematic situations in parenting.

EXERCISE

ROLE PLAY: FIRST WORKING DAY AFTER THE BIRTH

Some situations are suitable for a role play (see page 182).

Set the scene

Example

You have spent the first fortnight together at home, focusing on the baby, forgetting housework and the outside world. Today is the first normal working day for the father.

New father is still tired from the frequently interrupted night.

New mother says goodbye to him (in bathrobe, untidy hair, breastfeeding) with the words: 'When you come home tonight the flat will be nice and tidy, I'll have a supper ready, we'll be back to normal.' She thinks: I'll wash my hair, finally get into clothes . . .'.

New father comes home in the evening totally exhausted. The flat is littered with soiled and washed, but not yet dried baby clothes, there is no supper ready, new mother is still in bathrobe, unkempt and pushes their baby into his arms saying 'There, you can have your baby.'

The couples play the scene from here. He comes in through the door, she pushes the child into his arms. What could he do or say, to do justice to his own needs, but to her needs as well?

What could she do or say to do justice to her own needs but to his needs as well?

What needs has the child in this situation? Is there a solution that can be satisfying for all three of them? (Again each pair can find their solution, the one that's individually right for them.)

EXERCISE

THE FIRST WEEK AT HOME WITH OUR NEWBORN BABY

(Small group work see page 175.)

Helps towards a concretization and planning of everyday life after the birth.

Task: collect all possible fantasies and register them under one of the two following headings

Pleasant	*Unpleasant*
Visitors, Flowers, Celebration Getting to know the child Choosing a name etc.	Sleepless nights, sore breasts, sore perineum, Piles of dirty or not yet dry washing etc.

Gather and discuss all the pleasant and unpleasant fantasies in the large group. Maybe participants see the future situation as too rosy or too black, you can put it in still more concrete terms with the next exercise.

EXERCISE

QUESTIONNAIRE: DIVISION OF EVERYDAY CHORES

Visualizing the first week at home with your newborn baby?

Chores to be done	Who will do this?	I am happy with that	I am not happy with that
– changing baby's nappies			
– bathing baby			
– dressing baby			
– attending to baby when she cries			
– holding, carrying baby			
– attending to baby at night			
– cooking			
– shopping			
– washing up			

– tidying home
– vacuuming
– laundry – washing
               ironing
               folding away
– cleaning bathroom
– cleaning kitchen
– writing birth
  announcements
– phoning friends
– entertaining visitors
– caring for older siblings
– caring for pets

This could be filled in first individually (back to back) then compared and adjusted according to individual compromises, either in the class or as homework.

You can then discuss in the large group the solutions they found or are stuck with.

In the large group you can then work out a couple of general points for everybody to take home with them and to follow up on. Think which can be done to make the first few weeks easier:

Being specific in your request

– ask friends and relatives not to let the phone ring longer than three times but to ring back half an hour later — or consider buying an answering machine. Nothing is more nerve-racking than breastfeeding, bathing or settling the baby with the phone ringing on and on.
– ask somebody to deal with your washing in the first week or two. (take it away and return it ironed and folded – it is despairing to see mountains of washing piling up and for some reason never getting dry fast enough to make room for the next load) unless you have a tumble drier.
– ask various people beforehand to bring a meal or a cake when they come to visit you. Prepared meals will be a great boon. Store them in the freezer if you have one. Breastfeeding is hungry work, so it helps to have nourishing snack foods around too.
– ask specific friends and relatives to help with older siblings, take them to a playground, to their own homes, to the zoo etc. This will give them a treat and give you space to be alone with the newborn for a couple of hours.

It is very valuable to stress the importance of organizational details. It makes life so much easier. Make sure participants dare to ask a specific person for a specific task at a specific time:

Ann will come on Wednesday and collect the washing
Pat and John will come on Friday and bring a meal

Mum will come on Tuesday and bring various cakes to last a week of visitors
Hatty and Mark will take Elaine out for the day on Monday etc.

Encourage the participants to go further than just think:
'Who could I ask?
but to plan: 'Who *will* I ask?' and to actually do it. For some groups it's even important to clarify '*Who* will ask?' (the husband, his sister and his mother, or the wife, her sister and mother-in-law?)

If there is little awareness on how much life will change with a newborn, you can introduce the following exercise.

EXERCISE

TIME CAKE

Ask the participants to draw a large circle and divide it into 24 segments (cake slices).

The segmented circle represents the 24 hours of the day.

Suggest that everyone individually fills in the segments.

How many hours a day do they spend on: (average)

Sleeping/Eating/Earning a living/Gardening/Cooking/Cleaning the home/Laundry/Bodycare/TV/Reading/Sport/With friends/With partner/Alone/Other?

After they have filled in an average day ask the participants to draw a second circle and incorporate into this second circle the amount of time they visualize needing and wanting to spend with the baby:

Changing nappies/Breastfeeding/Preparing feed and bottle feeding/Carrying the baby around/Cuddling, Talking, singing with the baby, and then to see how much time is left for their other daily activities from the first circle. What has to be reduced or stopped completely. Within the couple relationship or with another woman in a 'woman-only class' they can compare and possibly make amendements to their second circles.

The discussion in the large group usually shows the grave difference between first and second circle for most women (her day should have to have at least 12 hours more, to still fit in all she would want or need) as opposed to the little changes most men make from one circle to the next (they might sacrifice half an hour TV here and an hour sport there to be with the baby or to help with the washing up).

What is gained though if we once again discover that the women take most of the load, it leaves both sexes angry, but helpless. Instead of or (if you think the 'time cake' is a necessary 'shock treatment') after the time cake exercise invite participants to the following.

EXERCISE

PLAN OF AN AVERAGE DAY

The aim of this exercise is *not* to develop a strict plan that has to be followed, but simply as an example to practise ways of communication and solution finding. And to become more and more aware of the situation as a parent with a newborn child and all the needs involved.

Hand out large sheets of paper divided lengthwise into three columns: She We He. Ask the participants to take down minutely an average day *without* a newborn baby, leaving lots of space for him/her, as they are doing so. Couples can work on this together, creating a picture of an average day, consulting each other as they fill out the respective columns.

Example

	She	We	He
6am			gets up goes jogging takes a shower gets dressed
6:15	gets up does some exercises		
6:30	prepares breakfast		
7:00	takes a shower gets dressed	have breakfast read newspaper	goes off to work
7:15	clears breakfast away		
7:30 etc.			

When everybody has completed the graph, just leave it aside for a while and introduce a large group discussion, gathering all the possible needs of a newborn baby on one placard and the needs of parents on another.

Put these placards up, visible to all and ask them to now fill the gaps on their day planner with the time to be spent on the baby's needs (first placard), keeping their own needs (second placard) in mind.

Partners do this jointly, reflecting:
  – what can we change in our present routine to fit our baby in?
  – who does which tasks?
  – what can we still prepare before birth?
  – which people can we ask for support?

EXERCISE

IMAGES OF IDEAL FATHER AND IDEAL MOTHER

Rosary (see page 173).

This exercise could be practised in various variations, each one will yield different aspects and insights.

1. two women together: an ideal mother . . .

   two men together: an ideal father . . .

   participants express their wishes and ideals about how their own mother/father should have been. What sort of mother/father they wish(ed) to have themselves.

2. heterosexual pair group (not one's own partner though), so that each can try out expressing ideals, without upsetting one's own partner.

   The woman – using the rosary method – tells the man in the pair group what an ideal father is for her.

   After a few minutes he gives feedback on how he feels, being confronted with these demands for high standards.

   Then the man tells the woman in the pair-group how he imagines an ideal mother to be, and the woman will give feedback after a few minutes.

   It is often easier to accept the feedback from a stranger than from one's own partner, where it is so much more emotionally loaded.

3. as in 2, but within the pair relationship

4. as in 1, 2 or 3, but with the variation that the woman imagines herself to be a man and says what 'his' ideal of a mother is and the man imagines himself to be a woman, saying what 'her' ideal of a father is.

   This last variation often brings a lot of insight and understanding for the wishes of their partners.

Needs of the parents

Parents who don't allow themselves to feel their own needs and deny themselves the satisfaction of their own needs for love, support, space, mothering, etc., will have difficulties in the long run, in being aware of the needs of their children, and be able to accept them and to satisfy them. It is important that we become aware of our unconscious needs, to acknowledge them, to reduce and alter those we can let go of, and to satisfy those we accept with awareness.

Points to consider   ○ Subconscious motivations
○ Self worth without children

Besides the above mentioned basic needs that all parents have there is a multitude of unconscious needs that could get in the way of a healthy parent–child relationship:

- women may need pregnancy, birth and motherhood to suppress or live, explore and challenge their femininity.
- women may need birth and motherhood as an examination in which they want to prove their abilities, strengths, altruism, endurance etc. to themselves, their partner, their colleagues, friends etc.
- men might need children to prove their own creativity, productivity, masculinity to themselves and others.
- parents might need this particular pregnancy and timing of parenthood to solve problems in their relationship.
    - to get closer again (like in the beginning of the relationship or during the first pregnancy)
    - to stop the partner from leaving (guilt and responsibility)
    - to feel stronger (not so alone) in order to cope with separation.
- parents might need a child as a decision maker, so that a frustrating job can be given up without guilt, or so that the mother will stop developing her independence and stay safely with the father of the child.
- parents might need their children, to be loved by someone or to have someone who is dependent on them.
- parents might need their children to have a reason for going on living (life has become so meaningless to them, were it not for the children they would commit suicide).
- parents might need their children as an expansion of themselves.
    - the child is allowed all the things they were not allowed (wear nice clothes, go to dance classes, join a certain sportclub, get dirty, keep pets, be naughty)
    - the child should live parts that they were not able to live (learn an instrument, receive better schooling, be better at sports etc.)
    - the child lives parts of them that they cannot live (expresses instant and intensive feelings: anger, desire, love etc.)
- parents might need their children to gain freedom to certain activities they would not allow themselves otherwise (swing on the playground, roll down a slope, play with a railway set, pleasure they would not have without children).
- parents might need their children to feel feelings they would not allow themselves otherwise.
    - feelings of tenderness and love.
    - feelings of sadness ('poor children, they hardly see their father, as a cover up for the rejection and loneliness the mother feels inside).

- feelings of envy and jealousy, ('why does he have to watch TV now instead of playing with the children', as a cover up for her own desire: 'I want him to have time for me').
- feelings of greed ('why does granny have to buy herself that new hat, instead of buying the grandchild the longed for tracksuit?' even if we would never ask for anything for ourselves, we can become demanding for 'our children's sake').
- feelings of confidence (suddenly we can say no to someone, or touch that spider, where, with no-one but ourselves to care for, we would not have dared to do so).
- feelings of pleasure (the cuddles, the closeness and laughter, seeing a bird again for the first time, sensing the earth, the grass, watching the clouds, anything takes on new meaning with a child).

In order to gather and discuss those needs in the large group it might be stimulating to ask participants to reflect on their individual needs for a few minutes. You can ask them, to divide a sheet of paper in two halves and write on one side everything they need from having a child, on the other side everything they want from having a child.

You could use this as a lead in to a large group discussion (nobody *has* to read out what they wrote down, but *can* share what they want to share!), or you could offer a pair exercise where they can sit with someone of their choice and talk about their needs and wants in more detail and openness.

In classes with couples it can be meaningful to form a women's group and men's group after everybody has written down their own needs and wants.

REFLECTIONS   Gathering and presenting the needs and wants of mothers and those of fathers separately, can lead to a very stimulating and valuable discussion in the large group.

The point of 'parents needing a child as decision maker' usually raises an important discussion.

Are we ourselves important enough? Do we really need a child, a pregnancy to finally follow our needs? Points to consider:

○ Self worth without children: to be able to get in touch with their ability to be happy, to have a meaningful life, to feel and express their feelings and to have pleasure whether or not they have children. With all the above mentioned points it is quite easy to point out how much unhappiness we can bring about in our families, if we need our children to live for us.

○ Sacrificing one's own interests
'I have done all that for you.' But have we really done it for them? or used them to do something for ourselves? [If we really

like our job, do we have to give it up just because we will have a child? If we really don't like our job, can we allow ourselves to give it up and don't need a child just for that!]

○ Preventing our own development through becoming a mother. Some women are scared, to make that next step in their career, because they don't trust their own ability. Because they are frightened by the challenge and the changes that would bring about, they opt for the 'safe way', getting pregnant! That prevents them from having to make the next step now, be it a change in their career or relationship.

It is not only the men who want to keep their women in dependence by giving them a baby! It is often the woman who are quite happy not to have to tackle the next step in their personal development.

But that's another important area to look at.

Does becoming a mother really mean a stop to personal development?

There is so much challenge and personal growth in parenting, probably more than any other job can hold, if it is only used.

○ The belief that the baby might rescue the relationship.
    If either of them fears that she might be leaving him if she gains further (material) independence through her job, then stopping work and having a baby will alter nothing. Either material and identity independence is of no importance to the relationship, so being a parent won't change anything – or it is of importance and being a parent will only increase the desire to gain it and thus threaten the relationship even more. If either of them fears that he might be leaving her be it for need of freedom or lack of responsibilities, the same applies.

It always boils down to the fact that happy and content families cannot come about through partners and children fulfilling each others' needs. Only if the parents individually, as woman and as man, lead a happy and fulfilled life, a happy family life can come about and a happy and content child can grow up.

○ I am the creator of my own happiness.
    I am responsible for my life. No one else is.

    If we need our partner or our child to bring happiness into our life it usually doesn't work out. This is not because our partner or our child lacks the ability to bring us happiness or has the power to withhold it from us, but because *we* lack the ability for our own happiness.

This is not a free ticket to egotism:
Your happiness is your problem so I can be as cruel or unresponding as I like.

If we choose to be friends with someone, to live together, there is now a joint venture to be taken care of. Now it is the happiness of our friendship or our marriage that we are both responsible for, not just one of us.

This mutual co-operation is there in the parent–child relationship too. Both are making an effort to make the relationship work. The parents giving attention to physical and emotional needs of the child. The newborn baby by rewarding with softness, innocence, total trust and by guiding with screams, whimpers and facial expression to even better understanding.

Later on as the child get older he or she learns that everybody has obligations. It learns to help (and it wants to as well!) with little chores. It learns to respect the parents' needs and space. It gives pleasure, love and trust. It has an inbuilt desire to do so.

Parenting fails, when either parents don't give their share to the mutual relationship or they take over too much, that the child unlearns to give his or her own share. It is the children who experienced either too little or too much parenting, who will grow up into adults who are unable to take responsibility, either for their own life or for a joint venture like a friendship or marriage.

○ Which values, beliefs and experiences of their childhood influence them now in their parenthood.

Each person brings his/her own family history into the relationship. These different backgrounds suddenly take on new meaning when one becomes family oneself. It is valuable if partners become aware of their difference and learn to communicate them before the baby is born.

In small groups participants can share their experience of being a child and what their family situation was like.

You could try the four corner method (see page 181) and participants can choose the theme they feel most connected to.

EXERCISE

FOUR CORNERS: FAMILY BACKGROUND

Group 1   What was allowed, what was forbidden in our family
Group 2   How were conflicts solved in our family
Group 3   What was the role of the mother/the father in our family
Group 4   Which events from my childhood would I like my children to experience too. Which events from my childhood would I like to avoid passing on.

After sharing the results from the small groups in the large group you could conclude the session with one of the following exercises.

EXERCISE

PASSING ON OF VALUES

Aim of this exercise is to:

– Become aware how many different values exist. How they can burden and limit us.

– Become aware and choose those values that are of individual importance.

– Realise that the partner might have different values.

– Discuss this difference, to adapt and/or possibly 'delegate' the passing on of certain values to the partner.

Do a brainstorming with the whole group collecting all possible values participants hold, on a big sheet of paper. Include values they want to pass on to their children and values they think should be passed on.

Then everybody on their own chooses nine of these values and numbers them in order of importance.

Couples then talk about which values each of the partners chose.

After the exchange, each partner should try individually again, to strike the three least important values off his or her list and to renumber the remaining ones, and talk to partner again.

Individually again, everybody reconsiders his or her list discarding a further three; exchange again with the partner.

The last step is for everybody to formulate a sentence, a motto for themselves (grammar is of no importance) and to share this motto with the whole group.

It is important to remind the participants how their values might be in conflict with the individual being of their child: their individual child might not thrive on the values they have chosen. It is important to know one's own values (rather than acting unconsciously upon them) but to remain flexible. Values, like everything else, need reconsidering: possibly changing, possibly re-affirming.

EXERCISE

FLOWER PETAL EXERCISE

Draw and cut out cardboard flowers with five petals. Use three different colours of cardboard.

Give one flower to each participant (different colours for men and women) and ask them to fill each petal with the value/ability they would most like to pass on to their children. The value or ability they find most important should be written in the middle of the flower.

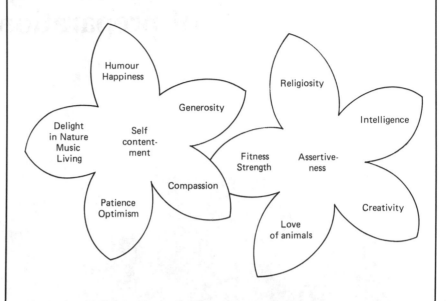

After filling out their flowers, the couples turn to one another, compare their flowers and are now handed a different coloured flower that they are asked to fill in as a couple. Which values can they agree on as the most important ones that they will jointly pursue? For example: Can the woman accept that her partner wants to pass on religiosity although that is not one of her values.

Parenting goes far beyond feeding or changing methods, interrupted sleep and piles of washing. It is important to remind parents of that.

You could bluetack the flowers on the wall or use the info-line (see page 176) so that everybody can look at all the flowers, before they take their flowers home. Maybe to hang up in the nursery, as a reminder of what it is really all about.

27 Daydreaming – a method of preparation for birth

As our bodies need a fever or an eczema every now and then to process certain 'toxins', so does our psyche need dreams and/or daydreams, sometimes even nightmares, to process and eliminate 'psychic waste-products'.

Many people tend to suppress fever and diseases through the use of drugs and so deny their body the possibility of expressing and healing itself. In a similar way many suppress their dreams and daydreams, forgetting them or distracting themselves when frightening thoughts come up.

As antenatal teaching is not intended as a form of therapy, the aim of guided daydreaming here is not to evoke particularly scaring situations and images. It is important, that the suggestions and the language used to give them are neutral but allow for the possibility that anxiety can come up if it is there.

The course facilitator needs quite a lot of sensitivity. If you feel uncertain, leave it. Guided daydreams are not a necessary part of birth preparation. If you like the method, don't just take the following daydreams as they stand. Find your own words, your own language. It is important that you yourself are in tune with your own words. Only then can you use daydreams effectively.

Guidelines for using daydreams

1. Be clear about your reasons for wanting to use daydreams

○ What do you want to achieve with this daydream?
○ Check, whether the content and the phrasing of the daydream are in tune with your aims.

2. Give suggestions through questions and images, not through descriptions of images

The less concrete the suggestions the better,

For example:

You arrive at the hospital . . .
What is happening first . . .?
How are you welcomed there . . .?

not:

You arrive at the hospital . . .
A midwife with a friendly smile leads you into the preparation-room.

3. Keep the daydream relatively short (max. 15 min. with preparation)

It is better to separate different subjects:

Example

- Start of labour
- Arrival at the hospital/routine measures
- First stage and transition
- Second stage and first encounter with the baby
- Coming home from the hospital
- Three weeks later

4. Leave enough time between the questions and suggestions

Insert pauses in the right places.

Example

Now go back in your thoughts (short pause to allow a separation from the preceding images) to the moment (*) when you felt the movement of your child (*) for the first time (pause).

(*) no pause as the suggestion is not completed.

5. Remind the participants by means of your language that they are in a daydream

Example

'Now imagine . . .' or 'See what comes up in your mind . . .' or 'What might you be feeling'

not:

'What are you going to do now?' or 'What are you doing now?' or 'What do you feel?'

6. Stay within one tense

Don't jump from past to present tense or from present to future tense or vice-versa.

Example

'Now imagine you feel the first contractions . . . how might you feel them? . . . What do you envisage yourself doing?'

not:

'Now imagine that contractions begin . . . what did it feel like? . . . What is the first thing you will do?'

7. Address the participants in one mode only   'You' works best. 'We' or 'I' make people feel uneasy sometimes.

8. Don't use indirect negative suggestions   *Example*

'Just let your thoughts come' or 'Now return your attention to your body.

not:

'You don't have to think too hard about it.' or 'Now leave your child, come back to your body.'

9. Don't use direct negative suggestions   *Example*

'Are you able to talk about it?',

not
'How was it for you, did you become aware of anything?',
'You can't talk about it.'
'You didn't feel anything.'

Ways of working from a daydream

1. Just leaving it at that   Leave it at that, as something to take home

2. Flashlight   With an invitation to share the mood or the content of the daydream.

3. Reporting to the large group   The participants report their dream images in the large group. No discussion or interpretation takes place.

4. Talking about the dream in pairs	A talks for five minutes. B just listens, then says how he/she perceived the basic feeling of the dream. Now reverse roles. (After the pairwork, flashlight in the large group.)
5. Talking about the subject of the dream	For example, filling in gaps in people's knowledge after discussing a daydream about birth. Or after a daydream on the theme of 'the ideal parent' gathering and discussing the images, by making graphs, displays, or lists.
6. Spontaneous sharing	No instructions after the daydream; everybody can talk about whatever she/he wants and as much as she/he wants.
7. Evaluating the dream reports for yourself, as the teacher	Was the child desired? What are the fears/tendencies? What is the level of knowledge? (Not to be shared with the group directly)

Different ways of tuning in to a daydream

In a new group with participants who are not used to relaxation and meditation, a preparatory exercise such as a simple relaxation should be done. If necessary follow this with questions: 'Did I speak loud enough?' . . . 'Did I speak slowly enough? . . .'Is everyone in a comfortably relaxed position?' . . . 'Does anybody need a cushion?' After this is sorted out, give another brief relaxation as an induction and only then begin the daydream.

If daydreams are offered more often, the induction can be shorter. The participants will be able to tune in to the daydream mood more easily after some practice. A daydream in deep relaxation is an aim in itself and can be as healing as a dream.

In our work, however, a guided daydream is not necessarily a daydream with 'deep relaxation.' One can just ask the participants to sit comfortably, close their eyes, listen to questions and let the answers come spontaneously. This is a good way of tuning the participants in to a subject in order to discuss it later in the large group, or have it worked on in pair- or small groups.

In this case the guided fantasy is a means to an end, a 'guided reflection' rather than a daydream.

The above guidelines cover both guided daydreams and guided reflections.

Physical relaxation as induction

Find a comfortable space for yourself . . . sitting, lying, on your side or on your back . . . whatever you like . . . take your time . . .

Allow your eyes to close . . . and really feel inside yourself what your body wants to do . . . how your body wants to lie . . . help yourself with pillows to support your head, your knees, your back . . . wriggle around . . . experiment with slightly different positions . . . really feel your way into the position in which your body wants to be in . . .

And then just let go . . . just relax . . . feel the contact with the floor, the cushions which support you . . . feel where your clothing is touching you . . . feel your hair in your face . . . just be aware of all the sensations your body is feeling . . .

Observe your body's breathing . . . just let it happen, don't alter it . . . just be aware of it . . . observe which parts of your body are moving with each breath . . . notice how deep down in your body you can feel the breathing . . . just observe it and let it happen . . .

Your body is taking care of itself . . . you don't need to do anything . . . all your limbs are relaxed and heavy . . . you don't need to hold them up in any way . . . your body is supported and feels heavy . . . rooted in the floor and in the pillows . . .

If you still feel tense anywhere in your body, just focus on your outbreath for a while . . . with each outbreath, let the tension melt away . . . breathe out . . . let go . . . breathe out . . . let go more . . . give a little sigh with each outbreath . . . blow the tension away . . . really feel, how your body is getting more and more relaxed . . .

At this point you can either introduce a guided daydream straight away or fit in a relaxation of the mind. After the daydream conclude with words like:

. . . And just stay with that as long as you want . . . and when you feel ready . . . slowly . . . move your fingers and toes . . . move your hands and feet . . . stretch your arms and legs . . . take a deep breath in and sigh out . . . yawn and stretch yourself . . . wriggle your back and neck . . . get movement back into your whole body . . . and when you feel ready . . . slowly . . . open your eyes . . . and gradually come back into our circle and sit up . . . still feeling in touch with your body's needs . . . get into a sitting position that's really comfortable for you . . . take your time

Relaxation of the mind

Now that your body is relaxed:

Observe the thoughts that come up . . . look at them and let them pass . . . don't hold on to them . . . don't intentionally continue the thoughts . . . just let them happen and watch them . . . watch them like you would watch a movie . . . images pop up and fade away . . . new thoughts come . . . let them go . . .

Your mind is taking care of itself and of you . . . just like your lungs do . . . like your heart does . . . you can rest . . . you don't have to consciously breathe nor pump blood through your body . . . you don't have to think . . . just let it happen . . . just rest and let the thoughts pass by . . .

At this point you can either lead over to a guided daydream or conclude with the last part of the physical relaxation. (see above)

Short induction for a guided daydream

Find a place for yourself in this room . . . lie down or sit down . . . whatever feels more comfortable . . . take your time . . . stretch a little . . . yawn and sigh . . .

Let go of any tension inside you . . . let your body find a position in which you can be relaxed and soft . . . let yourself be supported by the ground beneath you . . .

Let your breath flow freely . . . if you want to: take a deep breath and sigh . . . allow yourself to be entirely relaxed.

Examples of guided daydreams

JOURNEY INTO THE PAST – THROUGH THE PREGNANCY

And now I'd like to take you all on a little journey into the past . . .

You don't have to force anything . . . nor to make up anything . . .

Let your thoughts wander where they will.

I'll give you a little guidance and you just observe what occurs in front of your inner eye . . .

Let us begin with the present:

Try now, with your eyes closed, to let an image come of this room and of yourself within it . . . sitting or lying . . . as you are . . .

Be aware of how you see yourself and how you feel yourself . . . and then let the image go again.

Go back in your thoughts to the beginning of today's class.

As you settled down in this room, how did you feel then . . .?

Are there images and thoughts in your memory?

Just let them be . . . regardless of what is there . . .

Now go slowly back through today . . .

What are the things you have been doing . . .?

How did you feel this morning . . . when you got up . . .?

Just look . . . which memories and feelings arise before your inner eye . . .

Don't force anything . . . just look what comes up . . . as if you were watching a movie.

Now go further back . . . through the last week . . .

Important or small, forgotten events might appear . . . moments when you were entirely yourself . . . situations when you were . . . very different to now . . . just see what comes up . . . trust your own images, even when they seem to be unimportant.

Take it all in and then let it go . . .

Now go back in your thoughts through the last weeks . . . don't hold on to a thought . . . let an image, a memory appear . . . look at it and let it blurr again . . . don't produce memories, just look what comes by itself . . .

Everything is equally important . . . don't select . . . observe your thoughts, wherever they go . . .

And now go back in your thoughts to the moment when you felt the movement of your child for the first time . . .

What did it mean to you . . . what are your memories and feelings . . .what were you doing when you felt the movement of your child for the first time . . . what else was happening at that time . . . in your job . . . in your life . . .?

Allow the images and memories to appear . . . don't hold on to them . . . let them go . . . and let other memories come up . . .

Now go back with your thoughts even further . . . to the time when your tummy became round . . . what was your life like then . . .? When your tummy began to slowly get bigger what did this change mean to you . . .?

What memories and feelings come up . . . of events . . . talks . . . remarks . . . which had to do with the growing abdomen and the child . . .?

Just look what is there in your memory and wants to come up . . . take your time . . . don't force anything . . .

And then let this memory fade again . . .

Go even further back to the beginning of the pregnancy . . . take your time . . .

What was happening during those first months and weeks . . .?

Your job . . . your relationships . . .

What memories and images come up . . . of situations . . .
talks . . . plans . . . feelings . . . which had to do with your new
state . . .?

And now go back in your thoughts to the moment when you first
realized that you were carrying a child . . . or had fathered
one . . . What was your life like then . . .?

What feelings and memories come up . . .?

And now let go of them again . . .

And now come slowly back to the present, to yourself, as you are
here in this room, sitting or lying . . .

How have you been today . . .? What memories and thoughts
about your pregnancy are there now . . .? What is important in
your life now . . .? Allow yourself to know it . . .

And now sigh . . . yawn . . . stretch . . . roll over onto your
side . . . come slowly back to the group . . . very slowly . . . take
your time . . .

JOURNEY INTO THE FUTURE – THROUGH THE PREGNANCY

Be aware of yourself, as you are, lying in this room . . .

See yourself with your eyes closed . . . your position . . . your
clothes . . . the room you are in . . . the other participants . . . and
now imagine how in a little while you will stretch . . . how you'll
sit up again . . . and how you'll come back to the group . . . You
don't have to do it now . . . just imagine it . . . imagine that this
class is over . . . and you go home . . .

What will you be doing tonight . . .?

See yourself getting ready for bed . . . imagine how you will feel
tonight, at the end of this day . . .

And now imagine what you will be doing tomorrow . . .

What plans and ideas come up . . .?

What feelings come up when you look ahead at the coming
week . . . things you still have to do . . . people you are going to
meet or who you would like to see . . . events that might
happen . . . just let your mind wander forward in time . . .

Now imagine that you are at full term . . . you are expecting your
baby any day now . . .

Imagine how you might feel . . .

And now imagine that labour is starting . . . what do you think it
will feel like . . .? How do you guess it will happen . . .?

Will it be day . . . or night . . .?

Will you be at home . . . or somewhere else . . .?

Will you have somebody around you . . . or will you be alone . . .?

How might it be for you . . . will the waters leak or break, or stay intact . . .?

Will you have strong contractions at once or will it all start slowly, almost imperceptibly . . .?

Where will your men be when labour begins . . .?

Will you have to be called . . .? How do think you will feel . . . how will you react . . . when it is really happening . . .?

What do you see yourself doing . . .?

Stay for a while with the images . . . and then when you feel ready . . . come back to the present, to the class . . . to tonight . . . with several weeks still to go before your baby is due . . .

Now yawn . . . stretch . . . sigh . . .

JOURNEY THROUGH PREGNANCY – PREPARATION

This is not a daydream as such, but a very relaxing way to impart or take in knowledge.

I'd like to take you now on a journey through your pregnancy so far . . . so that as men you can also make contact with your baby, and, as a couple, you can make contact with each other.

It would be good if the women would sit on the laps of the men.

Men, find something to lean your backs against. Place your hands on the abdomen of your partner or on her sides if you prefer. Make yourself as comfortable as possible, so that you can both relax . . . you may find it easier to relax if you close your eyes.

Now breathe deeply several times [the facilitator does this herself] . . . and with each outbreath feel yourself melting even more deeply into the ground beneath you . . . letting go of any remaining tension . . .

check once again that you are really comfortable, and if necessary, shift a little until you are . . . let your breathing become deep and calm . . .

Now tune in to your baby . . . perhaps you can feel it moving right now . . . perhaps it is quiet.

Stay aware of your child now, as we begin the journey.

JOURNEY THROUGH PREGNANCY – VARIATION A

About every 28 days an egg matures in the ovaries. In the middle of the cycle, about 14 days before the next menstrual flow, this egg is released into the abdominal cavity and caught by the Fallopian tube. The egg then travels down the Fallopian tube.

It is only during this time that the egg can be fertilized by meeting a sperm. The sperm penetrates the egg and both cells merge. This allows the creation of the genetic code which is specific to and determines the development of the child.

On its way to the uterus the fertilized egg divides into more and more cells, so that it soon looks like a blackberry. This cluster of cells – your growing child . . . will have reached the uterus within a week there to nestle in the lining.

Your child is enveloped by an amniotic sac, which is filled with amniotic fluid. It grows, protected by the permanently renewed fluid. The placenta forms, and provides your child with oxygen and nutrients through the umbilical cord. The waste products of your child are eliminated the same way.

Let me tell you of some of the important steps of development that your child has gone through:
 – In the 3rd week heart and brain begins to form.
 – In the 4th week the nervous system, the genital organs, the skin, the bones, the lungs, the arms and legs, the eyes, ears and the nose start to develop.
   The heart of your child began to beat steadily.
   From that time on the official name for your child is 'embryo'.
 – In the 2nd month your child already looks like a small human being.
 – At the end of the 3rd month all the inner and outer organs develop. In the following months they are only further refined. The sex is recognizable. Your child dared its first movements, although you probably do not feel them.
 – In the 5th month your child already has hair on its head. Actually the whole body is covered with fine down.
 – From the 6th month on the contours of its body can be felt from outside and the physician/midwife can feel the position of the child. The skin is covered with an impermeable protective cream, the eyes can open, eyebrows and eyelashes grow.
 – In the 7th month your child already weighs about four pounds. Beneath the wrinkled skin fat develops and your child becomes plumper. If your child should decide to come into the world right now, it has a very good chance of surviving. However, most babies have just discovered how to suck their thumbs and are preoccupied with that.
 – In the 8th month your child weighs almost 5 pounds. The fine down disappears and the lines in the palms of the hands and in the soles of the feet develop.

– In the 9th month its home becomes almost too narrow for your child. The time approaches when she can no longer be nourished sufficiently inside you. Your child will have to leave its present home. The uterus has prepared for that by contracting every now and then during the whole of the pregnancy. You might have noticed that, especially in the past few weeks. Your tummy hardens as the uterus contracts. This can occur several times a day and yet it doesn't mean that labour has begun. When the contractions come more often and more strongly or when you feel a pull in the sacral area or in the tummy then your child is 'engaging'; finding its position for birth. Usually the head is pointing downwards, but it might also try to get out buttocks or feet first. Sometimes it will change position again and again. Then, one day, the contractions become more regular, longer and stronger, the pauses between them become shorter, and your breathing begins to change. Then you know that the cervix is opening to become your child's gateway into the world.

However, we are not that far yet. The cervix is still closed and your child has still some time to grow inside your abdomen. Maybe, you can feel it moving right now, or maybe it is quietly enjoying your attention.

Stay for some minutes with your child . . . and then come slowly back to the group.

JOURNEY THROUGH PREGNANCY – VARIATION B

Your babies have now developed so much they could live outside the uterus. This has been the fastest phase of development in their lives. I'd like to take you back to the beginning of this phase.

Through being together with your partner the egg and the sperm could meet and merge. Think back now, of the origin of your child . . .

The fertilization of the egg took place without your knowledge as did its wandering through the Fallopian tube and its nesting in the uterus. Here the child found its home for the next nine months. – When did you first think that you might be pregnant? – How did you react to this thought? – Did you trust your own inkling?

In the meantime the fertilized egg has nested firmly in the lining of the uterus. It developed quickly. The amniotic fluid and the placenta developed to nourish your child during its stay in the uterus. Now the pregnancy could be established for certain. – How did you feel with this knowledge? – Did it affect your relationship? – What new feelings came up in you?

Let us go further along in the course of your pregnancy. All the outer and inner organs of your child were developed; it was already so big that your belly began to round. One day you felt your child moving. – What feelings were triggered by this new awareness of your child?

Your abdomen is now getting bigger and bigger. Your child is always present to you now, whatever you are doing. You are learning to handle this new sensation. In which situations do you feel uneasy with your abdomen? – Can you cope with it? – Are there times when you like your belly or even enjoy it? – What sort of experiences have you had?

How does your abdomen feel now at this moment?
Can you feel your child inside?
Is it kicking firmly or is it moving gently?
Maybe it is sleeping or sucking its thumb, or drinking from the amniotic fluid, or peeing into it.
Stay focused on your child for a few more minutes . . . and then come back to the group . . . wriggle and stretch . . . and open your eyes.

TUNING IN TO THE BABY

This guided imagination is especially good for a mothers' class. You'll have to alter the text if you teach couples, in order not to exclude the men.

Roll over onto your side and curl up like a baby inside of the womb . . . and just feel yourself in this position . . . relaxed . . . supported . . . your breathing, your heart, your mind taking care of you . . . your body is cradled and cared for . . . you don't have to do anything . . .

Just imagine how it feels for the baby inside . . . feel what this baby wants . . . what it needs . . . get an image of what the baby looks like inside the womb . . . what it might want from you . . . feel, what you, just you, can give to this baby . . . and then feel, what you need for yourself . . . what you want from this child . . . feel, what this, your baby can give to you . . .

And be aware also of the exchange that is happening betwen you . . . hormones, chemicals, blood, oxygen, nourishment . . . you are giving to the baby all it needs . . . and the baby is producing hormones that you need to keep the pregnancy going . . . just feel the intimate contact between you . . . feel your baby moving inside you . . . vigorously, as if enjoying the extra oxygen it receives while you are relaxing . . . or quietly, relaxing with you . . .

Just enjoy the presence of two beings in your body . . . separate identities . . . and yet very, very close . . . feel how your body is

warm, warming and being warmed from inside . . . and just stay
with that as long as you want . . . and when you feel
ready . . . wriggle and stretch . . . slowly . . . and come back to the
group.

HOMEBIRTH – PART 1: START OF LABOUR

Imagine that the time has come. Contractions have started and
you know that labour is beginning.
- where do you imagine yourself to be?
- what do you imagine yourself to have been doing? – Is it day
  or night in your fantasy?
- are you at home or somewhere else?
- how do you visualize labour beginning?
- do the contractions start slowly and build up gradually?
- or are they strong and powerful right from the start?
- has the mucus plug come out? (In your fantasy, did you
  notice?)
- how?
- is the amniotic sac still intact?
- how do you expect things to go?
- what do you see yourself doing first when you realize that
  labour has begun?
- how might you feel?
    rather anxious or composed . . .?
    rather tense or joyful . . .?
    rather full or hungry . . .?
    rather exhausted, tired, or fresh and strong . . .?
- what sort of mood do you imagine yourself being in?
- what do you imagine yourself doing during the first minutes
  and hours of labour?
- when do you ring the midwife?
- would you rather be alone, or would you like to have
  someone else around you?
- who would you like . . . your partner . . . the
  midwife . . . friends . . . your children? . . . now that labour has
  begun . . . what do you imagine your partner to be doing . . .?
  how do you think he or she is feeling . . .?
- and where is the midwife . . .? what is she doing . . .?
- what would you like her to be doing . . .?
- how are your older children responding? (What do you
  imagine them feeling? What do you see them doing?)
- how do you imagine the labour progressing from this time on?
  How long do you expect it to last?
- what do you see yourself doing during the hours of the first
  stage?

– who is there in the house . . . and in the room in which you
    see yourself?
– what's the feeling in the house?

In your fantasy look around in the room you have chosen to give
birth in.
    – is everything comfortable, prepared and well-arranged?
    – is there something missing in the room or in the atmosphere?
    – what is needed to make things easier and more comfortable?

HOMEBIRTH – PART 2: FIRST STAGE

Now imagine that the birth began already some hours ago. The
contractions are frequent and more intense.

As the contractions get stronger and more intense how do you
feel?
    – how do you think your child feels as it experiences the
        contractions?
    – how do you think your partner feels?
    – how do you imagine yourself coping with the intensifying
        process?
    – where might you be?
    – pacing to and fro? leaning against a wall or on some
        furniture? in close physical contact with your partner or
        rather on your own? . . . Standing . . . lying . . . sitting?
    – do you imagine the midwife to be there by now?
    – what do you expect of her in this phase?
    – what happens in the hours of the advanced first stage?

What is your fantasy?
    – will you want to eat or to drink, to strengthen yourself?
    – will you still feel **OK** about going to the toilet or would you
        rather have a bed pan so that you don't need to leave the
        room or the bed?

Imagine that you are experiencing strong and regular contractions
with short pauses in between.
    – would you like to lie in a bath . . . or get some fresh
        air, . . . or have a massage?
    – would you want frequent examinations so that you know how
        far the cervix has opened? Or would you rather be left in
        peace?
    – what do you think will do you most good . . . feel best?
    – how might you handle the last hours of the first stage?

HOMEBIRTH – PART 3: SECOND STAGE

And now imagine that the cervix is entirely open. The first stage is over and the 'real' birth begins.

How might you feel?
  rather relieved
  or excited . . .?
  rather anxious
  or composed . . .?
  rather tense
  or joyful . . .?
  rather full
  or hungry . . .?
  rather exhausted
  or fresh and strong . . .?

What do you see yourself doing in the second stage:
  – will you change your position?
  – what position do you imagine taking?
  – will the midwife be in command or would you rather listen to yourself?
  – will you follow your own pushing urges or will you hold your breath and push as much as possible?
  In your fantasy how do you experience the contractions during second stage?
  What do you imagine your partner feeling?
  How will your child feel – will it be pushing to come out or be pushed to come out?
  How long will it be until you can see and touch the head of your child?
  What sort of co-operation will take place in second stage?
  How will it feel as the force of your uterus gradually pushes your child out?
  And how will you feel in those minutes when your baby is gliding out of the birth canal becoming ever more visible?
  Head . . . shoulders . . . arms . . .

HOMEBIRTH – PART 4: BIRTH OF BABY

And now imagine that your baby is born.
  – what might happen during the first minutes?
  – what is your baby doing?
  – what is your partner doing?
  – what is the midwife doing?
  – what are the other children/people in the room doing?
  – and where are you?
  – are you standing, sitting, squatting, lying?
  – how do you imagine that to be?

– are you holding your child in your arms or is your partner
  holding it – or the midwife?
– how are you feeling now that your child is born?
  rather relieved
  or excited?
  rather anxious
  or composed?
  rather tense
  or joyful?
  rather full
  or hungry?
  rather exhausted and tired
  or strong and fresh?
– how are you and what do you imagine doing during the first
  minutes and hours after the birth?
– first give birth to the placenta?
  . . . being stitched?
  . . . eating and drinking something?
  . . . nursing your child?
  . . . bathing your child?
  . . . taking a shower yourself?
  . . . sleeping, resting?
  . . . watching and caressing your child?
  . . . hugging and kissing your partner?
  . . . phoning your parents and friends?
  . . . celebrating?
– which of these or other things will you do first, second,
  third . . .?
– do you imagine the first hours to be quiet and calm or rather
  gay and noisy like a party?
– do you imagine the room to be cosy, the lights dimmed, or
  bright and well-lit?
– what do you imagine the midwife will do?
– will she retreat immediately?
– will she bath your child and take care of you?
– what role and what activities do you expect of her?
– how might your child feel in the first hours of its life outside
  the womb?

THE FIRST ENCOUNTER WITH THE BABY

Now imagine the birth, the physical labour is over.
There is your child . . .
  – how do you imagine this moment?
  – how do you imagine your first encounter with your child?
  – how will you feel?
  – how do you imagine your child?
  – who will be holding it or where will it be lying?
  – how will it be for you . . . for your child . . . during the first
    minutes of its life?

– what do you want from this first encounter?
– do you have any specific wishes for these first minutes?
– is there anything you fear when you think of the first minutes
  of your child's life . . .?

Now breathe deeply . . .
let go of your wishes and fears . . .

Breathe deeply again, breathe out . . .

We can talk about them later . . .

First come back to yourself . . . into this room . . .
give yourself a stretch . . . roll onto your side . . . and come
slowly back up . . .

COMING HOME FROM THE HOSPITAL, FIRST CHILD

Now imagine your child is born – some hours or days ago – and
you come home from the hospital.
  – how do you imagine your coming home after this great event?
    Your child is still very small and tender.
    Everything is still new . . . a bit strange.
    Maybe you are exhausted . . . maybe quite fresh . . . maybe a
    bit excited.
    You are bringing your child home . . .
     What are your fantasies?
  – how could it be?
  – what does your home look like? Look around – in your
    mind – is anything different from usual?
  – what does it feel like? Inside you and around you?
  – what is it . . . that you want from your partner for this day,
    this moment?
  – what's the first thing you will do after coming home? lie
    down? tidy up? receive visitors? Make phone calls?
  – how do you imagine your child behaving in his or her first
    hours at home?
  – how do you imagine your homecoming from the hospital?

And now breathe deeply . . . breathe out . . .
give yourself a stretch . . . wriggle . . . yawn . . . sigh . . . and come
back to the group.

Examples of guided reflections

HOW DO WE FOLLOW OUR IMPULSES?

Find a place for yourself, lie down or sit down so that you and your body feel comfortable . . .

Close your eyes . . . breathe deeply . . . and sigh if you want . . . allow your body to be soft and relaxed . . .

You are going to go on a little journey through the day. Just receive the questions and let the answers come up spontaneously.
- what did you do this morning when you got up – did you follow your impulses or did you follow your reason?
- when you met somebody: Did you want to talk or rather be silent? Did you follow your impulses or did you act against them?
- at lunch: How much and what did you want to eat and what did you really eat?
- during the day: What did you intend to do and what did you actually do?
- when you came into this room: Where did you want to sit and where did you actually sit down?
- what did you mainly follow today?
  Your impulses . . . your reason . . . your feelings . . . your needs or the needs of others and the outer circumstances?

Now breathe deeply . . . breathe out . . . wriggle and stretch . . . sigh and yawn . . . and come slowly back to the group.

TRUST AND MISTRUST

Feel inside yourself . . .
- which are the situations and the people you trust?

Now feel who you trust as far as the birth is concerned.

Who do you trust most?
- the hospital, a certain doctor, doctors in general, a certain midwife, midwives in general?
- yourself? Do you trust your knowledge or rather your body or your instincts?
- your partner? Do you trust his or her knowledge or rather his instincts? Which ability in him or her do you trust particularly?
- what or who else do you trust?

Now allow yourself to know who you don't trust when you think of the birth?
- which doubts and questions come up?
  Just allow yourself to feel the distrust.
- let yourself know what or who you don't trust. And then breathe deeply and let go of it.

Breathe deeply again . . . stretch and wriggle . . . lets talk about it in the group.

CONTROL AND SURRENDER

Every birth — not only the first one — is an entirely new experience.

How do you usually react, when you have to face something unknown — do you tend to be curious, anxious or aggressive?

How do you usually cope with unknown situations:

Can you go into them trustfully, or are you more likely to be cautious and tense? Or do you take the lead immediately so that you are in control of the situation?

Now imagine yourself responding to the birth?

Are you likely to want to control everything or can you imagine following your body and your instincts?

Might you be afraid or too shy to make noises, to show your feelings, to let yourself go?

Have you ever been in a situation in which you trusted that it was alright to let yourself go or rely on someone for support . . . and then felt that this trust was badly received or disappointed.

How did you respond to this?

Do you believe that self-control has a generally positive or negative influence in the birth process?

Breathe deeply again . . . stretch and yawn . . . take your time . . . and slowly return to the group.

28 When you have reached 'the end'

If you feel 'rock bottom' at the end of a class session and want to explore for yourself what triggered your feelings of despair, anger, helplessness or whatever it might be, try the following:

REFLECTION
- what do I feel right now?
- are there any physical symptoms. (Shivering? Headache? Are any parts of my body tense?)
- what happened (at the moment when I began feeling that way)?
- what else have I felt today? (feelings and experience I had before the event in class)
- what does this remind me of?

Just letting yourself know what is actually going on around and inside you not only relieves the feeling of despair but makes it concrete enough for you to deal with it further. If you experienced a conflict situation in one of your sessions/classes, that you were unable to solve at the time, you might want to ask yourself the following questions:
- who were the people involved?
- what do I know about them?
- what did they say/what did they not say?
- what was my instinctive reaction?
- what was the mood of that class generally (and at that moment)?
- was the conflict situation representative in any way
  - for the group?
  - for individual participants?
  - for myself?

- how do I feel about my own life at the moment?
- what connections can I recognize?

But do remember also the image of the suitcase that is mentioned at the beginning of this book: the suitcase that you can sort out over and over again, getting more and more clear about its contents, the weight gradually lightening, as you are able to distinguish between the essential and the superfluous . . . and the possibility that you can simply leave the suitcase behind and walk off – free!

APPENDIX

Examples of course structures
    Course for couples
    Course for women only
    Fathers' evening
    Weekend courses

Setting your house in order — a metaphorical exercise

Tips and guidelines for expectant parents
    Last few weeks of pregnancy
    Spontaneous start of labour
    Induced start of labour
    Early first stage of labour
    Late first stage of labour
    Transition
    Second stage of labour
    Third stage of labour

Tips and guidelines for birth attendants

An ideal image of antenatal and postnatal care and how birth could be in hospital

Credo

My beliefs

Appendix

Examples of course structures

Course for couples 8 sessions weekly   7.30 to 10pm.

This version is one example of a course that runs over 7 weeks in the last two months of pregnancy with a 6-week gap before the 8th evening: the reunion after all the babies are born.

The course is designed so that the vital information and exercises for birth are covered in the first 4 sessions, in case of one or two babies coming early. The last 3 sessions offer space for exploring the issues further, more time for discussion as well as preparation for parenthood.

From the second evening onwards, each evening starts promptly at 7.30pm. with a 'How is everybody?' with time to tell the latest news and developments and to ask questions relating to the current situation, allowing late comers to still be in time for the first exercise. At the end of each evening there is space for 10—15 minutes to wind down, to say goodbye to the participants, perhaps to answer individual questions, and if necessary, extend the session right up to 10pm.

Each of the issues or exercises introduced, can be followed up by a flashlight, feedback or discussion depending on the needs of the group.

As you will see, this course syllabus uses only a fraction of the exercises introduced in Parts I and II. Exercises can be mixed to suit your needs and the requirements of each individual group.

Course outline 1. Session

   o Introducing myself, my basic beliefs and aims
   o Body awareness I: Here and now

○ Self-introduction of the participants in a circle
  Name, expected date of delivery, home or which hospital? Their
  expectation of birth, their experience of pregnancy so far
○ Reflection: Introduction as a 'little birth'
○ Eliciting expectations for this course: snowball method

Break

○ Using visual aids to give an overview on the last few weeks of
  pregnancy and the normal birth process
○ Basic information and exercises to aid the relief of aches and
  pains that can accompany pregnancy
○ Eliciting and giving information about the start of labour
○ Guided daydream: Journey through pregnancy (into the past)
  to point of conception
○ Sharing the experience of the daydream in the large group

Homework: Body awareness I, at any time and place

2. Session

○ Body awareness II: Bodyparts
○ Information: Normal process of first stage of labour
○ Likely interventions, pros and cons
○ Possible methods of pain relief, pros and cons
○ Touch relaxation

Break

○ Basic information on breathing during labour
○ Breathing rhythms for first stage of labour
○ Stress exercises to simulate labour
○ Guided daydream: Journey through pregnancy (into the fu-
  ture) visualizing the start of labour
○ Group discussion on theme of daydream
○ Any questions that are left over

Homework: Applying rules for breathing in everyday situation

3. Session

○ Body awareness III: Floor, clothing, air, wellbeing
○ Information on transition
○ Discussion and exercises on the themes of fear and pain
○ Information on possible complications

Break

○ Breathing rhythms for transition
○ Pair exercises, sensitizing the couple to one another
○ Guided reflections, trust and mistrust
○ Discussion and sharing, open questions

Homework: finding some positive phrases for birth (self affirmations)

4. Session

- ○ Body awareness IV: Inner space
- ○ Exercises to loosen the pelvis and pelvic floor
- ○ Information on second stage
- ○ Breathing rhythms for second stage

Break

- ○ Talk and discussion about the postnatal period: how do we want to receive our babies
- ○ Information on breast feeding
- ○ Guided daydream: First encounter with the baby

Homework: to try out breathing rhythms while passing a motion

5. Session

- ○ Body awareness IV: Inner space (shortened version)
- ○ Reading of one or two birth reports
- ○ Pair exercise on pain: 'to open and to accept help'
- ○ Stress sequence as labour simulation
- ○ Guided reflection: Control and surrendering

Break

- ○ Preparation for parenthood (Questionnaire, group work, pair work, roleplay)
- ○ Pair exercise: 'To trust and to dare'

Homework: to use touch relaxation and the trust exercise with each other

6. Session

- ○ Body awareness IV (even more shortened version)
- ○ Guided daydream through labour in three or four parts with intervals between to fill in gaps of knowledge, have time for questions, repeat a breathing rhythm or touch relaxation exercise
- ○ Centring exercise, glass sphere

7. Session

- ○ Body awareness IV (shortened to 2 minutes)
- ○ Dress rehearsal

Break

- ○ Awareness exercise: Moving like a newborn child
- ○ Time for questions, sharing problems, last tips
- ○ Guided daydream: Coming home from hospital

8. Session (after the birth).

○ Reunion, with the babies
○ Birth reports
○ Celebration
○ Food and drink
○ Questions
○ Sharing
○ Tips

Course for women only

8 sessions, weekly   7.30–10pm or 9.30–12noon.

Classes for women only can run along the same lines as couples classes with little adaptation only: the content need not differ; the emphasis does though.

In couples classes I want to stress the importance and beauty of sharing birth and parenthood, raise inspiration and interest in the couples, quite inappropriate for most single women who would simply be reminded of their loss or would not feel addressed, if their values differ.

It is generally more satisfying for everybody if separate classes for women only are offered.

Single mothers or women whose partners won't be there for labour and birth have different needs, that cannot be catered for in a mixed class. Plus they could raise feelings of unease, envy, fear etc. in the couples present. Feelings that might be important for them to deal with, but not in the context of an antenatal class.

Catering for the different needs of single mothers does not dictate a course structure necessarily different from the one above. Even the pair exercises are just as effective if women do them together to explore their own trust, sensitivity, awareness or whatever the exercise is intended for.

What does need to change, however, is the facilitator's own approach and how she deals with the themes and questions that come up. In classes for women only the participants are often a lot more open and intimate with one another which offers different opportunities to the teacher.

In that sense it is important to resist the temptation to replace a class for 6 couples with a class for 12 single women. It is not just a question of how many comfortable seats your room offers but how many pregnancies and life stories *you* can contain in any one class.

The other question is am I better suited to teach couples, or single mothers, at different phases of my own life?

I might go through a rocky patch in my own marriage and feel quite hostile towards men in general. I may not trust that they are fully capable of real sensitivity and care. With an attitude like that I am not likely to inspire trust and co-operation in a couples class.

Or I might feel totally happy in my own relationship. Treasure and enjoy the sharing of pregnancy, birth and parenthood and feel nothing but pity for 'all those women who have to go the path alone'. This attitude is unlikely to inspire confidence and joy in motherhood in a women's only class.

I might just be deeply hurt by my own man's infidelity and full of anger about mistresses who 'get themselves pregnant to try and catch a married man.' An attitude that would stop me from giving real warmth and care to some of the participants in a women's only class.

There is the other side to it too.

I might just have reached a phase in my own relationship where things have gone stale, there is some disappointment . . . but still it seems alright. Teaching a women's only class in that phase of my life, might just rock the boat as the independence and strength of some of the women in the class inspires me to look at my own life more clearly.

Teaching antenatal classes can change our lives in more than one way. It can make us broody, it can inspire us to try again with our man or another man, etc. Teaching is never just one-way.

Ideally we have experience of all aspects: of happy marriage, of being left or of walking out, of feeling jealous, lonely and depressed, of feeling strong, independent and joyous . . . so that we can be sister and friend to single mothers and couples alike.

Most of us though will have to be content with the awareness of where we are at and what our needs and gifts are at any given moment, and to use them accordingly.

Fathers' evenings

Most women-only classes include one or two fathers' evenings. These sessions are often quite tense for everybody.

Some women are worried that their partners might be bullied into being there at birth or being helpful in the weeks after, and that this will only increase their defensiveness. They often fear that the man's indifference will change to rejection, whilst at the same time hoping that he will 'miraculously' discover his interest in birth and family life.

Most men need persuasion to come along to fathers' evenings. The facilitator is often confronted with defensiveness, indifference or superiority ('What's this all about anyway . . . haven't women given birth for thousands of years?'). On the other hand there are always a few who are sincerely interested in learning as much as possible, and who regret not having been able to attend a class for couples. All this puts a lot of stress on the facilitator who feels she has to put on a specially good 'show'.

My own antenatal teaching has changed a lot since I started and I have altered many of my beliefs about it. In the beginning I saw myself as the all-important person in the lives of the couples coming to me. I would not admit new participants halfway through a course because they would have missed half of *my* teaching and would not know what it was all about. I am now much more relaxed. I have realized that they often go to other classes as well, read books, and generally have quite a lot of information.

So when I hear other teachers talk about fathers' evenings I suspect that they maybe carry similar beliefs. They sigh about all the information that needs to be packed into one evening: 'How can three hours be enough?' 'I'll never get all that across.'

There came the point when, having up till then only taught couples classes, I took my first women's class. When I asked the women in the group whether we should have one or two fathers' evenings, the response was 'I'll be glad if he comes along to one.' Their main concern for the evening was to talk about postnatal depression, i.e. to indicate to the men that they would not be jolly and fit for a while after birth, and not cook a three-course meal every day after coming home from hospital.

I kept all that the women had said at the back of my mind while at the same time being aware that I did not want to appear to the men as a moralist in alliance with the women.

When the fathers' evening came I decided to hold a normal 8.00–10 class and to be as empty as I possibly could. By 'empty' I mean going unprepared, with no structure for the evening, but simply being available to the couples. To respond rather than to feed or moralize. I decided not to adopt the usual approach of starting when everyone was there and providing books for people to delve and withdraw into beforehand. Instead I began the evening when the first couple arrived.

After a chat about the weather and public transport problems I asked him how he felt about the hospital class he had been to, what had remained unclear to him, whether he had any questions left.

We were right in the middle of discussion and teaching when the second couple arrived. They listened for a while, and then I repeated the same question to the second husband. And so on. The whole two hours were filled with questioning and answering without any structure. Nevertheless, when I looked back on the evening, I saw that we had covered information about the labour process, had practised breathing and massage, had talked about the problems of adjusting to a newborn baby (i.e. the birth of the family) and a lot more.

Of course there were even more unanswered questions when we ended at ten o'clock, but I felt good about this, because I don't see my job anymore as giving all the answers, but in stimulating questions and involvement. Those men with further interest would be able to find answers from their wives or in the books that their wives read etc.

So for me, a fathers' evening is primarily an evening for discovering what interesting subjects pregnancy, labour and parenthood actually are. If I had attempted to give all the answers, the subject would have appeared closed, and the men would have shown no more interest than before.

Weekend courses   It is pleasurable to work for a whole weekend with a group of couples or women. The only aspect that is missing is the time to integrate the lessons into everyday life. A very important aspect in antenatal teaching. This is why, personally, I prefer either two weekends with a fortnight's interval or even better, four consecutive Saturdays.

Example:

1. First Saturday

  o Getting to know each other
  o Basic knowledge of the last few weeks of pregnancy and birth
  o Keep fit, awareness and centring exercises
  o Guided daydream on journey back through pregnancy
  o Breathing observation and awareness exercises
  o Exercises and discussion on trust, fear, pain or similar

2. Second Saturday

  o Information – on the different stages of labour
    – hospital routine pros and cons
    – medication pros and cons
    – possible complications

  o Further awareness and centring exercises (to intersperse the large Information part)
  o Breathing rhythms for the different stages of labour
  o Guided daydream on journey forward through pregnancy.

3. Third Saturday

  o Exercises and discussion on trust, fear, pain or similar
  o Stress sequence
  o Guided daydream on labour in three parts interspersed with
  o Awareness centring and sensitization exercises
  o Touch relaxation and massage
  o Time for questions, sharing

4. Fourth Saturday

  o Further awareness-, centring- and sensitization-exercises
  o Dress rehearsal
  o Preparation for parenthood
  o Guided daydream on first encounter with the baby
  o Information on breastfeeding
  o Discussion, sharing, time for questions.

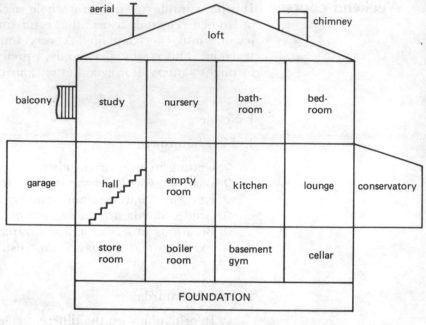

Setting your house in order – a metaphorical exercise

The various rooms and features of a house can be symbols for different aspects inside you. I would like to invite you to look at those step by step.

Environment   Everything which surrounds you. From 'political situation' right down to your 'work space'. How do you feel about the people and issues that are in your personal environment? Do you feel safe? What can you do to improve your environment? What images do you get when you think of your environment?

Foundation   Our basic beliefs and feelings, our relationships and framework of friends. How supportive and stable is the framework? How solid and deep rooted are your foundations? Can you build on your own trust and optimism? How integrated is your pessimism? What images do you get when you think of your foundations?

Boiler room   What is the source of your energy (money, anger, love, satisfaction . . .). What keeps you refuelled? What drains your energy in your life, your work? Is there enough energy left in you. Is there one central source of energy in your 'inner house' or are there separate radiators in every room? What images do you get when you think about your Boiler room?

Home sauna/
Billiard room/
Gymnasium

How well do you take care of your own body? What do you do for yourself to experience your strength and pleasure? Did you/do you do the physical exercises yourself that you suggest in your classes? How do you really feel about them? What would your imagined Basement room look like?

Store room

What information, memories and feelings do you store away unnecessarily? Keep checking whether your mental 'preserves' aren't out of date. Beware of mould (your own bitterness and doubts). How full or empty is your store room? Do you know what is in it? Does it need stocking up or clearing out? Do you spend a lot of time in it, sorting through your papers? (Preparation time for classes) or have you got it all handy anyway? What images do you get when you think about your store room! Could it be a utility or play room?

Cellar

How much space is there in you for your feelings? Is your cellar a dark room that you hardly enter or is it well lit and ordered? Are your emotions well kept in barrels, slowly maturing, or is there an uncontrolled fermentation process happening, ready to explode? What images do you get when you think about your cellar?

Hall

Do you take everything and everyone to heart or keep them at bay, or do you let issues and people come too close? Do you allow others to have a hall or do you go straight to their living room or even bedroom? Is your door tightly closed, easy to push open, wide open at certain times?
What images do you get when you think about your inner hall and front door? (Is there a back door where people can reach you more easily or 'get at you'?)

Empty room

Is there space inside you that is uncluttered that is open for new ideas, thoughts, feelings? Is there room in you without preset values, empty of personal objects(ions)? Are you easily influenced and fill any available space immediately with theories and structures? Can you allow one part of yourself to be unstructured, without imprint, just open. How big or small is this space in you?

Kitchen

How much nourishment can you give to others? Are you mothering, demanding, spoiling? Do you have set ideas about what is good for others? Are you an expert on nutrition? Can you encourage others to find out what is good for them – using your larder, your kitchen utensils? Are the 'meals' you serve delicate and thoughtful 'starters', solid, warm, rich stews or impressive sweets? What images do you get when you think about your inner kitchen and the 'meals' you serve?

Lounge This stands for issues of relationships, feelings, communication, sharing, exploring, discussing. How much space do you give for that in your work? How important is that in your own life? How much at home are you in your inner lounge? What images do you get?

Conservatory This can stand for pleasure, luxuriousness and enjoyment or cultivation, properness and display. What sort of conservatory do you have in your work? Do you allow space for pleasure? Do you believe experiences have to be difficult and painful in order to be effective? Do you believe real learning and change can come about through pleasure? How important is it for you that your exercises are aesthetic, your discussions harmonious, your classes beautiful? What images do you get when you think about your inner conservatory?

Bedroom That is relaxation, massage, breathing, intimacy, bodycontact, closeness, privacy, being with yourself. Do you allow yourself space for that? Or is it just important for other people, but gets neglected in your own life? How much are relaxation, massage, breathing, just techniques for you, to be learned before and applied at birth? How much are they integrated into your whole life? Is there a door from the bedroom to the living room (emotions) and to the conservatory (fun)? What does your inner bedroom look like? Lived in? Tidy? Uncared for?

Bathroom How much space do you have to pamper yourself? How luxurious, light and large is your bathroom? Is make up, outer appearances very important to you? Can you accept that inner beauty might be more important? Can you accept too that inner openness is more important than any stretching exercises, massage of nipples or pelvic floor? What does your inner bathroom look like?

Study How important are facts, studies, research-results in your life? How influenced are you by book-knowledge? How dependent are you or your course participants on the latest scientific results? What 'truths' does your study contain? Can you use your study as a space where you can be quiet and listen in to yourself? What is the image of your study?

Nursery   How much room do you give the child inside you? Are you in contact with your needs? Can you express yourself spontaneously and intensely like a child? Is there space for colour, toys, games, fun in your life? Is your nursery fully equipped, overflowing with things you hang on to from childhood or tidy, stripped to the essentials? Does your nursery leave space for the development of the individual (child) inside you? What is your image of your inner nursery?

Loft   Do you have space for superfluous things in your life? Do you have a space in yourself where you can go and hide? Do you have a space inside you where you can go and explore, finding new and long forgotten treasures? What images do you get when you think about your loft?

Chimney   Where do you let off steam? Is your chimney blocked, large enough, regularly cleaned? What does your chimney look like? Who or what is the chimney sweep in your life?

Aerial   Are you in touch with God, with a spiritual being that loves you and sends you energy and protection? Can you receive the energy and love that is around you in nature – plant, animal and mineral, stars, in other people . . . What does you aerial receive? Does it need adjusting, correcting?

Balcony   Do you have a balcony in your professional life, where you can be seen, where you deal with public relations? Are you really interested in improving the birth situation, or are you quite glad about the status quo, as it gives your role as antenatal teacher meaning and importance? What do you do on your balcony? Who can see you there? Have you got insight into neighbouring professions.

Garage   Is there a space in your life that enables you to get away from it all and do something completely different? Do you have a car? Is there petrol in the car? (Do you have energy left, if you have the time to get away)? Do you have the car keys? Or does somebody else hold the key to your happiness? Can you see yourself in the position of holding your own keys, available to you any time you want them and having enough petrol to go as far as you want? Do you waste a lot of your energy driving round and round or on escape attempts? Where would you really like to go? What is your image of the perfect break or holiday? You deserve it!

Tips and guidelines for expectant parents

Last few weeks of pregnancy

What is happening	Tips for the pregnant woman	Tips for husband/friend
○ Most women notice frequent contractions (Braxton Hicks Contractions) in the last few weeks, sometimes even coming regularly for a few hours. These contractions prepare the uterus for labour. ○ With each contraction your uterus feels hard and bulging. ○ Sometime in the last 4 weeks your baby will 'engage' into his or her birth position. That might lead to increased back ache, more frequent passing of water and irregular bowel movement but also less pressure on the stomach and easier breathing. ○ Some babies only engage with the start of labour. ○ Some women have more vaginal discharge than normal, sometimes pink or brownish. Should any bleeding occur notify midwife or hospital immediately ○ Sometimes the cervix is already several centimetres dilated, weeks before the baby is due and yet labour only starts on or after the expected date of delivery. ○ Some women have a spurt of energy a few days before labour starts. ○ Most babies are less active in the last few days before labour but if you are concerned about your baby not moving enough contact midwife or hospital immediately. ○ Some women lose weight spontaneously a few days before labour. ○ Some women have diarrhoea shortly before labour.	○ Ask your midwife or doctor, whether the baby is already engaged. ○ Try to relax with each preparation contraction (Braxton Hicks) so that you get a reflex going: contraction starts – you relax. ○ Experiment with different breathing patterns during those preparation contractions. Observe which pattern suits you best. ○ Prepare all necessities and 'extras' for home or hospital birth and for the time afterwards. ○ Put a plastic sheet under your bed linen in case the amniotic sac breaks to prevent the mattress getting soaked through. ○ Don't spend all your energy on housekeeping in case labour starts that day or night. ○ Follow your own needs and impulses those last few weeks. Sleep, rest, eat, move about, as little or as much as you like even if it is at odd times. Allow yourself to be pampered. This will help you to understand and respond to the baby's irregular and seemingly unreasonable needs. ○ Be open for anything. Even a well engaged baby can struggle out of an engaged position and turn breech or into posterior presentation and vice versa. Babies can even change position in First Stage of labour. ○ Try not to have any fixed ideas about what labour should be like, just stay with a trusting and positive attitude.	○ Warn those concerned that you will suddenly need one or several days off ('holiday') in the near future. ○ Prepare a list of all the phone numbers where you can be reached, should labour start when you are not around. ○ Prepare a list of phone numbers that you might need to phone midwife, doctor, hospital, grandparents etc. ○ Do a test drive to hospital, explore side routes in case of rush hour traffic. ○ Find out about parking possibilities near the hospital. ○ Plan or organize something pleasant to do on the evenings, weekends *after* the expected date. If the baby should be late in coming there is something else to look forward to.

Spontaneous start of labour

What is happening	Tips for the woman	Tips for the labour partner
o The amniotic sac might burst or leak, yet labour contractions could only start hours or days later. o The amniotic sac might stay intact until the end of first stage, unless it is ruptured at an internal examination. o The mucous plug that sealed the cervix might be discharged yet labour contractions could only start hours or days later. o It could also happen that you don't notice the discharge of the mucous plug or that it is only dislodged after you have had regular contractions for several hours. o You might have regular contractions for a day or longer without it being real labour. As long as contractions last 10–40 seconds without increasing in strength and length they are still preparation contractions, however frequent or regular they are. Once contractions are 50–90 seconds long, they effectively open the cervix even if there might be long pauses between them. o Every woman has a different pain threshold, yet experiencing the early contractions as very painful does not necessarily mean that the really effective later ones will have to be even more painful. You and your body might be more tuned in to the contractions by then and better able to cope with them. o You might not notice any painful contraction until you are well into First Stage and are suddenly surprised by very strong and frequent contractions.	o As long as contractions are not increasing in frequency and intensity continue your usual routine. o If it is nightime try to sleep a bit more or at least rest with a warm water bottle. Get up in the morning as for a normal day. Move about but don't do anything strenuous. Conserve energy for birth. o You can take a warm bath. This will either help you to relax and give you an additional rest or it might activate stronger contractions and get the process going. o If the amniotic sac bursts and a lot of fluid comes out in one gush, this is an indication that the baby's head is not yet or not anymore properly engaged. Call midwife or hospital and lie down until it is confirmed that there is no prolapse of the umbilical cord. o During the birth process your uterus uses all your energy and the stomach is slow in digesting. If you want to eat or drink, take easily digestable nourishment. Yoghurt, juice, herb teas. Don't take lots of honey or glucose as this might lead to a sudden rush and fall of energy. o Don't get excited too early. As long as you're not sure whether this is labour it probably isn't. o Follow your impulses. Call the midwife or go to hospital whenever you feel you want to. Trust your own urges.	o Don't forget yourself. Have a rest, eat and drink as long as you are not yet desperately needed. o Some women want to be left alone and just focus on their body. Just to have your nearby and to know that you are available should she need you, might be all that's required. o If wanted offer distraction and entertainment for the pauses in between contractions as long as she wants it (games, reading, TV, music, going for a walk). o If contractions are regular e.g. every 4 or 10 minutes, you could keep an eye on the watch and remind her $\frac{1}{2}$ a minute or so before the next one is due, so that she can prepare inwardly for it. o Remind her to breathe out and 'let go' with the start of each contraction.

Induced start of labour

What is happening	Tips for the labouring woman	Tips for the labour partner
o Sometimes it is considered safer for you or the baby if labour is started artificially. o After your arrival at hospital at the given date you will most likely have an enema, or suppositories, have a bath and maybe a pubic shave. At the internal examination the midwife or doctor will most likely pop the membranes of the amniotic sac allowing the waters to leak. o Sometimes this is enough to trigger contractions as the baby's head presses more strongly onto the cervix without the cushioning effect of the amniotic fluid. o Depending on the routine of a specific consultant or hospital you might be given a hormone to induce contractions at the same time as the membranes are popped or after a few hours or a day's wait. The hormones can be given orally as tablets or as a liquid or vaginally as a pessary or via a drip into the arm. o An induced labour is often experienced as being more painful and the onset is not as gradual as a natural labour process, although that need not be, as the amount of hormone given can be regulated to suit individual needs. Some hospitals/doctors deal more sensitively with that than others. o If your labour is induced it is most likely that your contractions and the baby's heartbeat is observed by a continuous CTG. You might also have a drip with a glucose solution so that your blood sugar level does not drop.	o Relax during and especially after the enema and the internal examination. o Don't hold any tension in your pelvic floor. o Refuse to be shaved. This is a totally unnecessary procedure whether or not you are induced. o Ask to be propped up with cushions. An induction is no reason to lie flat. o Try and get as comfortable as you can. Ask for help if you want to change position so that the wires of the CTG don't get disconnected or tangled up. Don't let that stop you following your impulses for a different position. o If you find contractions overwhelming let your midwife and doctor know. There is no reason why an induced labour should only last a certain number of hours. You can request that the drip be slowed down. Most likely your body has produced enough hormone in the meantime, so that your own natural labour could take over. o Inquire about the induction routine, this varies greatly. o Make an aware choice.	o Enquire whether you are allowed to be there from the beginning or only allowed in after induction procedures are completed. o If you prefer to be there from the beginning try and make this possible by talking to the staff or changing hospitals. She might need your closeness and attention during the induction procedures and while waiting for contractions to begin. o Once contractions start she might need even more attention and encouragement than for a normal labour as her body has to get used to, initially at least, artificially induced contractions. o Don't forget though, that it is her healthy body and self that deals with it, don't let her feel like an ill patient even though she is lying and connected to various bits of machinery. o Encourage and aid her relaxation between contractions, if she wants it – with the help of massage and touch relaxation. o Remind and encourage her to release tension with her out-breath, to sigh and groan, to let go of her anger, frustration or whatever she might be feeling. o Be totally with the labouring woman and don't pay too much attention to the machinery.

Early first stage of labour (1–5 cm)

What is happening	Tips for the woman	Tips for the labour partner
○ The muscles of the uterus tighten and shorten during each contraction, pulling the cervix upwards and relax and lengthen again in the interval betwen contractions.	○ Relax with and after each contraction and allow your own breathing rhythm to flow.	○ Encourage her. Trust and believe in her own strength. Don't pity her. Don't belittle her feelings.
○ The cervix gradually shortens and opens more and more.	○ Go to the hospital or call the midwife whenever you feel you want to.	○ Be sensitive to whatever she wants, distraction or rest in between contractions.
○ With each contraction the blood supply to the baby is restricted. This means less oxygen to which the baby responds with a drop of heart rate to make the little oxygen last longer. Frequent checking of the baby's heart rate allows the midwife to know how well the baby recovers after each contraction.	You might feel safer being within the hospital grounds walking around there, without actually going to the labour ward yet, especially if you know that the routine in the hospital of your choice is to speed things up if you get there quite early.	○ If necessary and wanted do most of the talking for her (admission procedures, explaining and requesting your individual wishes) so that she can concentrate fully on her body during contractions.
○ Contractions can come at varying intervals. Some women have contractions every 2 minutes, others every 4 or even 10 minutes.	If you get to the labour ward once your labour is well established, there is less likelihood of routine procedures that you don't need or want.	○ Remind her to go to the toilet every hour. A full bladder could press against the opening cervix. She might not feel the need to pass water as other sensations are much stronger.
○ It is possible that you might not feel any pain with the contractions until you are a few centimetres dilated.	If the hospital staff are open to your individual needs, go to the admission as early as your want.	○ If she has back ache give back massage and counterpressure. Check frequently where and how strong she wants the counterpressure.
○ Contractions can last 50 or more seconds. It is the length of the individual contraction not the frequency that influences the dilation of the cervix most.	○ Follow your body's needs regarding position, be upright and mobile as long as possible if that feels right to you.	○ Give as little verbal instruction as possible. You can guide and support her breathing and relaxation with touch relaxation and by emphasizing the outbreath yourself.
○ The contractions can be experienced as back pain, as period cramps, as warm orgastic rushes, as a mixture of all three.	○ Drink frequent sips of sweetened herb tea, juice or yoghurt to give your body the fluid and refreshment it requires, for if your urine is tested and your blood sugar level is found satisfactory this will avoid the necessity for a dextrose drip.	○ Whenever she loses her breath, breathe out audibly to encourage her to do so too, this will help her to again find her own rhythm.
○ Once in hospital or after the midwife's arrival at home the baby's heartbeat and the cervix will be examined and you might be given an enema or suppository.	○ Welcome and enjoy each contraction as positive work your body does for you. Don't fight your own process.	○ With each of her outbreaths you can stroke along her back, arm or thigh downwards, continue stroking her at this rhythm even if her breathing gets temporarily faster or erratic. This will help her to return to her own rhythm.
	○ Enjoy to be overwhelmed or enjoy to be on top of things, go with whatever is happening.	○ Keep checking with her what she needs, don't be disheartened if her wishes and needs change frequently or if she does not need you at all.
	○ Stay in touch with the signals your body is sending.	○ Relax! Take care of yourself.

Late first stage of labour (5–10 cm)

What is happening	Tips for the woman	Tips for the labour partner

○ The individual contractions last longer and are more intense. They are often, though not necessarily, more frequent than before.
○ If the first 5cm dilation took 10 hours this does not mean the next 5cm will take as long. Usually the first 3cm take longest and after 6cm dilation it can go very fast. Though: no rules without exception.
○ You might well want to accept pain relieving drugs at this stage.
○ You might be very tired and fall asleep between each contraction. Your uterus is working very hard and uses almost all your energy and oxygen supply.
	○ Follow your body's needs
	  – lie down, altering sides, to be really comfortable
	  – go on all fours to relieve back ache
	  – Keep walking about if that helps you to release excess energy.
	○ Take whatever position helps you to relax and let go. Any position or movement that is a strain for you wastes energy that your uterus could need now.
	○ The more relaxed you are, the more you give in to the contraction, the faster the cervix will open.
	Allow yourself to feel great love for your baby or partner. The cervix just slides open while kissing, hugging and exchanging loving looks and phrases.
	○ Watch the tendency to choose a position where it 'hurts less'. This might slow down the progress as you are not really letting yourself into the process.
	○ If you do find contractions unbearable it is especially important to breathe well as it will be hard going for your baby too.
	Accept pain relievers if you cannot cope with the intensity of pain. Do anything that will prevent you tensing up and fighting the process.
	Do everything that will help you release and aid your giving in to the process.
	○ If you have 'surrendered' to accepting pain relieving drugs, try and trick yourself: knowing that you will get something soon try just one more contraction without pain relief, and then maybe one more . . . and maybe one last one before you accept the drug.
	Quite often you can help yourself over a rough patch with this trick and may find that after those few contractions you actually can manage without drugs.
	Alternatively, you might suddenly find yourself being in second stage already, your 'giving in' having helped to speed the process along.
		○ Encourage and aid her focus on her own body.
		○ Encourage and praise her, there is progress even if she does not feel it. Talk to your baby in her womb. Coax it to come out.
		○ Many women forget in the intensity of the labour what it is all about.
		○ Let her feel loved and cherished. The baby is not more important than her.
		○ Observe her face, shoulders, hands, etc. Aid the release of tension with touch relaxation, refreshments, warmth etc.
		○ Help her into comfortable positions by arranging cushions or furniture or allowing yourself to be used for support.
		○ Offer drinks or moist flannels to suck (the lips get very dry).
		○ Refresh her face or hands.
		○ Don't say 'relax' but stroke the part of her body that is tense.
		○ Help her to look forward to the next contraction.
		○ Massage her back using counter pressure if this is needed.
		○ Accept, that she might not need or want any help or touch at all.

○ Unless you opt for an epidural in
early labour, there is the risk or
'chance' that you will ask for one
when you are 5–7cm dilated . . .
and end up being fully dilated by
the time the anaesthetist has set
up the equipment. Opt for Gas
and Air in late Second Stage.

○ If you do accept pethidine or
something similar, don't expect it
to remove the pain. Allow
yourself to float into the drowsy
state that it induces. If you fight
the effects of pethidine you will
only end up experiencing them
negatively. For more information
on drugs see Further Reading
(Chard/Richards and Inch, Sally)

Transition

What is happening	Tips for the labouring woman	Tips for the labour partner
○ Transition can last 2 minutes or 40 minutes. ○ Contractions and the intervals between them can be very irregular which makes it difficult for you to adapt and flow with them. ○ The cervix is almost fully dilated, maybe there is just on one side a small so-called 'lip' left. ○ The baby's head presses directly onto vagina and back passage and thus stimulates a pushing urge. ○ Your body receives contradictory messages: 'hold it, cervix not yet dilated' and 'start pushing'! Your body is in confusion and reacts often with shivering, vomiting, feeling feverish. All these are positive signs; your body is releasing blocked energy. ○ Most women want to give up at this stage, want to go home, want a general anaesthetic, just want to sleep, regret ever having wanted a baby. They might get very angry towards their man who fathered the child, towards the midwife who seems unhelpful. ○ This change of attitude is normal and a sign that second stage is almost there! ○ Some women don't have a transition at all, but move	○ Remember, though highly unpleasant, the signs of transition tell you that the birth is nearly there. Labour is soon over. ○ Try not to waste your energy on pushing, while the cervix is not completely dilated. ○ Bear down gently if you can't help it, without holding your breath. ○ Keep the supply of oxygen going, talk, mumble, sing just to keep breathing. ○ If you want to, use gas and air at the beginning of each contraction or throughout transition. ○ Don't ask for or accept any other drugs at that stage, as they would only start taking effect when you are in second stage and you might be too dozy to give birth and greet your baby consciously. ○ If that feels right, use a position where the pressure of the baby's head onto the birth canal is relieved, kneeling on all fours with your head lower than your buttocks, or lying on your side. ○ Let your body work for you. Accept the shivering, vomiting etc. gratefully. ○ Release any anger freely (holding back any feelings prevents you from opening). It is all right to	○ If wanted, help her into a position where there is least pressure of the baby's head. ○ Remind her that the signs of transition are positive, that she's almost there. ○ Let her know that you love her, that she's wonderful even though she might be really annoyed with you and show her unpleasant and dark side. ○ Don't doubt her ability to cope. Her body is prepared and really helps her though it might appear differently. ○ Be observant: what tenses and blocks her more; – is she wasting energy on bearing down prematurely? – is she getting all tense and tight, trying *not* to respond to the pushing urge? ○ Encourage her to let her body take over, not to strain or fight anything. ○ Accept her anger graciously as your part of bearing labour pains. ○ She might just cling to you for continuous support, literally sharing the pain with you, or she might not bear to have you near her. ○ Stay in touch with your own needs. This is an intense time for

smoothly from first to second stage.

scream and shout, everybody knows that this is transition and you are at heart loving and forgiving.

you as well. Be prepared for strong feelings in yourself too, let them out if you need to. But don't get stuck in them. In two minutes it could be all over. Let your feelings change with the flow yourself.

Second stage of labour

What is happening	Tips for the labouring woman	Tips for the labour partner
○ The muscles of the uterus do not relax in between contractions, but remain tight and short, getting even tighter and shorter with the next contraction. Thus the uterus gets smaller and smaller, gradually pushing the baby out. ○ It can only last a few contractions, but on average it lasts 30–40 minutes. ○ As long as there is progress and the baby's head is gradually more and more visible in the birth canal and the baby's heart rate is normal second stage can last two hours or more. ○ In some hospitals it is routine to complete second stage with a vacuum extraction or forceps if the baby is not born within a certain time. ○ The baby's head presses onto the back passages, so one sign of second stage is for women to think they have to pass a motion. It is quite normal despite enema or suppository that some faeces or wind is pushed out as the baby descends. The wall between vagina and rectum is stretched and very thin. ○ As the baby moves downward and outward through the birth passage – the vagina is and feels very stretched. This is a hot and tingly sensation (try stretching your mouth with your fingers). ○ It might feel as if tearing, the pelvic frame feels like bursting. Yet is is built to contain a baby and created to give way.	○ Be totally guided by your body as to when and how strongly you need to bear down. Let your body do the work and aid it by breathing well and focusing on opening and letting go. ○ If you push without a pushing urge you exhaust yourself unnecessarily, rob your body of energy and oxygen and put pressure on your perineum before it has sufficient time to stretch. ○ Don't worry if you pass a motion or break wind, it is totally normal in second stage. ○ Let yourself be completely relaxed, all the work goes on between your diaphragm and your perineum, everything else can be loose and relaxed, your face, throat, shoulders, arms, hands, legs. Let your uterus have all your energy. ○ If you want to or need to hold your breath for bearing down breathe in-out-in-out-in quickly before you hold your breath. That way you get more oxygen than with one deep inbreath. ○ Trust the power of your contractions. Trust your vagina and pelvic floor to stretch. Don't fight against the sensations. Be open for the birth of your child. ○ If contractions weaken and progress slows down or stops – change position from horizontal to vertical or vice versa, both changes can help. – move and circle your pelvis to loosen up.	○ If she wants to know tell her how much of the baby's head is visible or hold a mirror for her to see. Seeing the baby's head emerge with each contraction can give new energy. The baby's head always slides back a bit during the interval to release the pressure onto the perineum. ○ Some women like to have the head held during contractions. Maybe that helps them unconsciously to relate to the baby, who feels pressure on his or her head. ○ Whenever she arches her back remind her non-verbally by placing a hand on the small of her back to keep her back rounded. ○ Give praise and encouragement. Some midwives ask for and demand more and more pushing when she is already giving her best. Encourage her to focus on breathing and letting go and just trusting and following her pushing urges. ○ Talk about the baby, it is normal for her to forget what it is all about as her bodily sensations are so strong. ○ Maybe she wants a moist cool flannel on her forehead in between contractions or a kiss . . . Show her your love and care. ○ If you have to wear a face mask remember that your eyes can show all your worry, fear, disgust, especially as she can't see your

⊃ If you should need an episiotomy the perineum is cut during a contraction and you will hear, but not feel the cut. There will be a sense of relief and the baby will be born with the next contraction.

⊃ For some women the perineum is numb with pain as the baby's head passes through, others experience orgastic relief. Though the image of the many folds of vagina opening like the petals of a rosebud is a beautiful one, do expect a much more powerful experience than the image implies. Giving birth is not just a gentle opening. It is one body coming out of another body. It is two beings parting that have been very close for 9 months!

○ Your body will guide you when to push and when not to push as each individual perineum needs different time and incentive to stretch.

○ Even if the midwife insists on delivering you in a lying down or semi-sitting position you can still get up for a few contractions in between to aid the baby's descent with gravity and loosen your pelvis through rotation. After a few contractions you can lie down again so that the midwife can support your perineum and receive the baby in a position that is comfortable for her.

smiling mouth. Try to express warmth, admiration and encouragement through your eyes.

○ Using the touch relaxation-reflex help her to relax her pelvic floor.

○ Help her and encourage her into a different position if contractions weaken. This is the only time when you might have to be firm to suggest a different position as she might have reached the stage where she can't be bothered. Yet she will feel better for it, once you have helped her into the new position.

Third stage of labour

What is happening	Tips for the parents
○ The baby is born! There is an enormous sense of relief yet birth is not quite finished.	○ Find out abut the routine procedures your midwife likes to employ/in the hospital of your choice.
○ The uterus is still contracting, reducing in size thus expelling the placenta.	For example:
○ You might be given an injection to speed up the expulsion. Depending on consultant or midwife this injection might be given shortly before the birth of the baby.	Is ergometrin/symtometrin injected routinely.
	The only good reason for this is to finish the process more quickly. If you should need suturing it is awkward to wait for two hours for the placenta to be expelled.
With the 'help' of the injection the placenta will come out within 10 minutes. Without the injection it might come in the same time but could also take up to two hours, which is alright as long as there is no excessive bleeding.	Everything has to be seen in context. If you want to avoid getting an ergometrin/symtometrin injection it is wise to prepare your perineum during pregnancy with pelvic floor exercises and massage using Vitamin E to prevent a tear or a cut.
○ Once the placenta is there it is checked to see whether it is complete to make sure no pieces of amniotic sac or placenta remain trapped in the uterus, which is now quickly closing the cervix again.	○ Should the placenta be slow in coming, nipple stimulation (putting the baby to the breast if it is interested in sucking) or squatting over a bucket might help. If necessary plead with the midwife to be patient. As long as there is no excess bleeding there is no reason to pull or tug at the cord or knead the uterus from above, all this might only lead to a partial separation which would *then* cause more bleeding.
○ The postnatal contractions cause the uterus to further contract – once the placenta is expelled it is reduced to the size of a grapefruit within one hour.	
○ If you had an episiotomy you will have a local anaesthetic, so that you don't feel the repair. The suturing can take a few minutes or up to half an hour depending on the size of the cut or tear and the skill	○ Find out what your baby is likely to experience in the first hours after birth: When will the cord be cut?

of the obstetric staff. You do not need to be brave now, ask for another local anaesthetic if you feel the stitching.

○ Usually you remain for two hours after birth in the delivery room, you are washed, the baby is examined and put to your breast for the first time. The obstetric staff want to be sure that there is not too much bleeding, that the uterus contracts nicely and that your bladder is working.

○ Some women start shivering once it's all over, no matter how many blankets they have to keep them warm. It is a normal physical reaction to the strain of labour.

Will there be dimmed light? Who will be present? Pupil midwives? Student doctors? Will the baby be given to you? For how long? When will it be examined? By whom? Midwife? Nurse? Obstetrician? In your presence? Another room? On the delivery bed, so that you can be near? Will the baby be brought to a central nursery while you are tidied up, given to your partner to hold? Placed in cot? Is the baby bathed routinely? Who will bath your baby? Would you be allowed to hold him or her after the examination or bath? For how long? When and how will your baby be dressed? etc.

○ Be clear for yourself how you would like the first hours to be. Express your wishes clearly, before you register with a midwife or in a hospital, in early labour and at the actual time.

○ If you experience the shivering after birth an energetic foot and hand massage seems to help. All the blood is still centred around the uterus and needs to be coaxed back into the extremities. Maybe the shivering is aiding this distribution of the blood.

○ You can request to get up to have a shower and go to the toilet rather than sitting on a bedpan straight after birth. This will help to get your circulation going too.

Tips and guidelines for birth attendants

○ Remain relaxed yourself
Breathe calmly
When you feel any tension release it with the next outbreath.

○ Listen to your own body signals
Be aware of your own needs and satisfy them if possible (different position, food, drink, fresh air etc.)
It will benefit the labouring woman.

○ Keep yourself in the background
The labouring woman is the centre of attention, main sender and receiver of signals, and all her signals are important.

○ Be aware of what your eyes are communicating
It is easy to restrain one's voice, even manage a smile but do your eyes look tense, harrassed, rushed?

○ Be aware of whether the labouring woman blocks her own flow of energy
She may do this by tensing up, talking too much, frequent change of position, negative attitude etc.

○ Be aware of any interference with the birth process
Is the room too cold, the light too bright? Is there tension

between husband and wife, woman and doctor, doctor and midwife. Find the cause and aid its removal. After a clarifying talk the birth process usually picks up again.

○ Do not interfere with a normal birth process
No medical intervention if not absolutely necessary. With any disturbance of the birth process check first for non-medical causes. See above.

○ 'Shower' the labouring woman with warm and loving attention
And, if necessary, warm water (bath) so that she can let go and give in to the birth process.

○ Encourage the labouring woman to use her outbreath or release tension (do it yourself too!)
Encourage her to sigh, groan, whether the sounds be pleasant or racked with pain. Especially if you observe a tendency to make sounds on the inbreath, encourage her to give way to sounds on the outbreath. If you observe high compressed sounds (iii, eee) encourage her to make low open sounds (hoooh, huuuh, haaah) (see page 104).

○ Don't encourage self pity
Encourage the woman to be positive in her words and actions so that the process can flow. If there is too much sadness, anger, pain etc. to be positive, encourage the release of those feelings with words, sounds, hitting or squeezing a cushion etc. Once those feelings are released the birth process will flow better than before.

○ Be aware of areas of tension in her body (forehead, jaws, shoulders, hands, buttocks, thighs, toes etc.).
Stroke over or along the tense part with every outbreath of the labouring woman. Do it gently or firmly – whatever aids the release of tension best. Or encourage her birth partner to do so. With these rhythmical strokes you can stabilize (slow down or speed up) her breathing pattern, if she should temporarily lose her breath.

○ Let her know that seemingly negative signs are positive
Stronger more painful contractions, stronger more painful back ache, are indications that the birth process is making headway. Involuntary bowel movements or vomiting are a sign that blocked energy is being released (often necessary when the labouring woman was hanging onto a very controlled behaviour).

○ Stay in touch with your own feelings
Observe and follow your own instincts and intuitions, if something doesn't feel quite right to you.

○ Watch your own language. Choose words and phrases that encourage the woman to open and let go.
Example
Right: allow it to happen, let it come, give in to it, well done, lovely etc.
Wrong: pull yourself together, you can do better than that, you mastered that last contraction very well etc.

○ Remind the labouring woman of the baby about to be born
That is what labour is all about – without giving her the feeling
that the baby is more important than her.

○ Encourage a change of position if you sense its necessity but let
the woman choose one that feels really right for her – whether
she wants to be upright, walk around, lie, sit, squat, or kneel.
Make sure that her back is not arched and that she is
comfortable in whatever position she chooses. (See page 150.)

○ At the beginning of second stage
Tell her that her cervix is fully dilated and that whenever she
feels the urge to do so she can bear down. Do not encourage
pushing before she is ready for it. Encourage her to continue
breathing well, for herself and for the baby. If progress slows
down encourage a different position (see pages 151 and 153.)

○ Take your time and give the new family time with each other
after the birth of the baby. It is nature's way that the placenta
does come instantly.

Let nature take its course and interfere only when really necessary.
Further excellent guidelines for birth attendants can be found in:
Davis   'A guide to midwifery'
Flint   'Sensitive Midwifery'

See Further Reading page 296.

An ideal image of antenatal and postnatal care and how birth could be in hospital

ANTENATAL CARE

○ At every visit the woman and her pregnancy are regarded and
treated as individual

○ Every antenatal visit is an opportunity to encourage self-
awareness and self confidence:
– by asking questions and listening to her answer
How do you feel?
Is anything bothering you?
What do you need?
What would you like me to do?
– by using symbolic language which will help her to understand
her body better;
constipation: – what is blocking you in your life?
– what do you want to stop happening in your
life?
pregnancy nausea: what or who do you feel sick about?
high blood pressure: what or who is it that makes your blood
hot? etc.

○ No routine measures at intervention. Every measure that
becomes necessary is explained:

– Pregnancy is a natural process like breathing or digestion. As long as it is normal it does not need to be observed and controlled.

Some people like to know the exact amount of acidity of their stomach, the frequency of their breathing or the circumference of their unborn baby's head; others are disquieted by any check-ups or the examinations might even lead to complications. The needs of the individual are responded to. Each pregnancy is regarded as individual.

○ Every visit is an opportunity to encourage and intensify the pregnant woman's/couple's trust in the midwives and doctors.
  – the pregnant woman isn't patronized, but treated with respect.
  – negative comments ('this baby has got a huge head', 'I can't find the other leg', 'the placenta is very low lying' etc.) are not made unless it is really proven that there is a disproportion or a deviation from the normal. If there is, phrases as neutral as possible and the reasons for concern and for any necessary intervention are explained.
  – verbal or non-verbal questions or statements are noticed.
  – nothing is done without valid reason and explanation.

Nothing is a greater hindrance to the woman's ability to flow with her own birth process than her mistrust of the medical profession. She cannot open herself fully to the experience if she keeps worrying: 'What are they doing now?' 'Is that really necessary?' 'What are the side-effects?' etc.

BIRTH

First stage ○ The labouring women/couples arrive in hospital at the very first signs of labour if they so wish.
They do not need to fear any routine measures (enema, shaving, induction or acceleration, continuous fetal monitoring, etc.)
○ They can move into their birth room and make it comfortable and homey.
○ The room provides a small fridge for drinks, yoghurts, ice cubes, and teamaking facilities.
A cassette or record player
If that is not possible they can bring in their own equipment, as well as recorded music, games, pictures, flowers, nightdress, t-shirt, anything to feel at home even if they might not use any of it.
○ The birth room also contains
  – a double bed, so that the partner can lie down too if labour lasts for a long time

- a chair that can be easily used backwards too
- a comfortable armchair or rocking chair (for partner, midwife or doctor).
- two surfaces (e.g. chests for equipment) one chest height and the other table height for the woman to lean on
- a soft mat on the floor to kneel or be on all fours on (or a firm double mattress on the floor instead of a bed)
- pleasant pictures, curtains, wallpaper
- daylight and warm electrical lighting
- a bucket or large firm ball for the labouring woman to squat on
- a climbing frame on one wall, or a string with thick knots at various heights for the labouring woman to hang onto
- an inviting looking cradle to stimulate pleasant thoughts of the baby
- private toilet facilities with a large bath tub and shower
- a baby bath

○ The labouring woman can take any desired position and is, if necessary, encouraged to move about and try out other positions.

○ The midwife stays with the labouring woman/couple for as long as the couple want her there in the room (knitting or reading in the rocking chair in the corner), or she can leave the room for longer or shorter periods as the birth process and sensitivity to the couple requires.

○ The birth process is not unnecessarily disturbed, any equipment that might become necessary is stored next door or behind curtains.

○ The tasks of the midwife are:
  - to check the baby's heartbeat and gradual descent
  - occasionally to check dilatation of the cervix
  - to encourage and aid free movement of the labouring woman
  - to encourage and aid free-flowing breathing
  - massaging or encouraging partner to massage (if wanted and necessary)
  - to provide the right atmosphere for opening and relaxation.
  - to be aware of and deal with any possible disturbances:
    - her own restlessness, antipathy or negative attitudes (for example: this woman will never manage)
    - rigid attitudes of the labouring woman (for example: over-controlled behaviour, clinging into certain positions etc.)
    - negative attitudes of the labouring woman (for example:
    - self-pity, fear, anger, envy, disgust etc.)
    - rigid or negative attitudes of the partner (for example: overprotectiveness, talkativeness, self-opinionatedness, fear, disgust etc.)
    - relationship problems (for example: she can't let go while he is around, she feels/shows more pain than necessary for his sake etc.)

○ The labouring woman can make as much noise as she wants and needs.

Second stage

○ Only when necessary will a doctor come and aid the midwife.

○ Internal examinations to establish second stage can be omitted as the external signals are usually clear enough. Women can bear down as (in-)frequently and as early or late in second stage as they need to.

○ Women can choose any position in which they feel genuinely comfortable and in which the birth process is unimpeded. (For some women lying down might be better than being upright: aids letting go, relaxation, feeling more urge to push; for other women being upright is important and right – working with gravity, greater mobility of the pelvis, feeling stronger).

○ As long as there is progress and woman and baby are well, second stage can last two hours or longer.

○ The woman, her partner or the midwife can massage the pelvic floor with or without oil, as desired.

○ Protection of the pelvic floor is given by the midwife in any position.

○ The woman's breathing and pelvic mobility are more important than her bearing-down efforts.

○ An episiotomy is made only when absolutely necessary.

○ A vacuum extraction or forceps are only used after a change of position has been unsuccessful.

○ The baby is received calmly: movements and sounds are friendly (laughter or screams of delight sound different to the baby than loud harsh orders).

○ The baby is given to the mother and/or father straight away.

○ The removal of nightie or shirt and vest is encouraged to allow maximum skin contact.

○ No injection is given to speed up delivery of the placenta. As long as there is normal bleeding the placenta can take as long as two hours to come out. Steady pressure from above (small sandbag on tummy) or squatting over a bucket, nipple stimulation, patience, help most.

○ The baby is only bathed if it seems right and the mother wishes it. S/he is not to be disturbed in its first hours if s/he is fine just snuggled up with both or either of its parents or wrapped up warmly in a blanket.

○ The baby is not dressed in vest, nappy and clothing but wrapped in warm soft towels, enabling the parents to explore and touch their baby's body if they want.

○ The woman is encouraged to get up, go to the toilet, have a shower or is given a 'bed-bath' if she wishes.

○ The family spend the remaining day and night in the birth room. The partner stays there as well. Clearing up is kept to a minimum, the special atmosphere in the room just after the birth is treasured.

- The family is given time for themselves.
- Food and drink are offered.
- The family returns home the next day or moves into another similarly equipped room in the maternity ward. The partner and older siblings can stay there for the night too if desired.

Maternity ward

- Full rooming in is possible (for fathers too if they want to stay the night.)
- The baby stays day and night in the bed of the parents if that is wanted.
- The sleep of mothers and babies is not disturbed by cleaning, taking temperature etc.
- Babies who are taken care of in a central nursery are comforted by cuddling, carrying, rocking, gentle music or taped sounds of maternal heartbeat.
- The mother can be sure that the baby will be brought to her if she is unconsolable.
- Breastfeeding on demand is encouraged and aided, as long as there is no objection.
- Nursery nurses are consultants and helpers. Mothers and fathers call upon them any time they want help with changing nappies, feeding, crying baby etc.
- Maternity and nursery staff don't offer contradictory advice. Maternity and nursery staff encourage the parents' trust in their own actions and intuitive knowledge. Parents are given a guideline for helping themselves and taking care of the baby at home.
- Weighing the baby is not important as long as s/he appears to be thriving.
- Sore or cracked nipples are treated with natural remedies.
- Tea-making facilities and herbal teas are plentiful.
- The main object of staying in the maternity ward is for the parents to be encouraged to be in touch with and respect their own needs, to learn to become aware of their children's needs and to be able to satisfy them. The same applies to the postnatal visits of the midwife if mother and baby are at home.

> **'HAPPINESS IS BEING ABLE TO FOLLOW ONE'S IMPULSES SPONTANEOUSLY'**

Credo

I believe   in the god of S P R I N G T I M E
in eternal rejuvenation and change
in rebirth and life
in an energy that is so powerful that it can't but grow

I believe   in the god of S U M M E R
in the abundance of life
in joy and beauty
in an energy that is visible and can't but show itself

I believe   in the god of A U T U M N
in the letting go that follows every experience
in sadness and forgetting
in an energy that loses itself and can't but dissolve

I believe   in the god of W I N T E R
in the withdrawal into the below and beyond
in dream and death
in an energy that is inside and can't but understand

I believe   in the goddess of L I F E
who embraces and contains everything
who is all that is
all we can see and perceive and
all we cannot see and cannot perceive

I believe   in M Y S E L F
in my abilities, possibilities and probabilities
in all the energies within myself
in challenge and surrender
in my life
and that I can't
but be myself

I believe   that we create our own reality
that we influence it
by our unconscious wishes, fears and attitudes
that all that happens is connected.

My beliefs

These are my beliefs about pregnancy, antenatal teaching, birth and parenthood. All readers are invited to challenge, dispute or rephrase any of these personal beliefs.

PREGNANCY AND ANTENATAL TEACHING

I believe that

- the timing and length of a pregnancy is not accidental.
- All our symptoms (aches and pains) have a meaning, that our body wants to tell us something with them.
- Our body knows what it needs and that it asks for it (through tiredness, backache, raised blood pressure etc.)
- We – at least during pregnancy – should live according to our needs and only do (eat, sleep, work) what we really want to.
- Women can learn to listen to their bodies and react adequately to its signals.
- All complications (premature contractions, high blood pressure, etc.) have a meaning and that we could avoid or solve them if we gave attention to the individual attitudes and circumstances of the couple involved.
- Antenatal teaching could and will be superfluous
  - if the situation in society and antenatal care were changed in a way that women would be treated as individuals, that their body awareness would be trained and their intuitive knowledge would be trusted (instead of undermined)
  - if childbirth professionals would only interfere when it's really necessary
  - if women would not need to fight for their rights but could trust their midwives and doctors fully

I believe that

- Antenatal teaching should not result in women being better adapted to the hospital system, or being able to keep themselves under better control.
- Antenatal teaching should not result in inciting women against the hospital system.
- Antenatal teaching is meaningful as long as it fills the gap which the hospital system and our situation in society creates.

I believe that

- Men are just as strongly influenced by the situation in our society and have to learn again to become aware of their own instincts, to trust themselves and their woman.
- Men, as much as women, need antenatal teaching to be able to cope satisfactorily with the complex issues.
- Women could have sorted everything out before birth so that at the time they don't need to think, doubt and fight anymore, but can go completely with their body sensations and can rely fully on their man and childbirth professionals.

BIRTH

I believe that

- The time at which birth happens is not an accident but corresponds to the inner needs and circumstances of parents and child.

- Our body signals whether it wants to stand, sit, lie, eat, drink etc. and that we can rely on these signals.
- Any dogma is bad, whether it is the routine use of pethidine or the routine use of squatting or bathing the newborn baby. Every woman and child should be attended to and cared for individually.
- All the symptoms (posterior presentation, vomiting etc.) which might occur during birth have a meaning and that we should listen 'within' to understand what our body wants to tell us.
- All complications are meaningful and correspond to the attitudes and circumstances of all concerned.

I believe that
- Some newborn babies want to die and are prevented from doing so.
- Some newborn babies have an incredible life force and survive defying all adversities.
- Nothing happens by chance.
- It is for a reason (maybe unknown to her) that a woman, chooses a particular hospital, and 'ends up' with a particular midwife or doctor.
- We are never at the mercy of 'reality' but that we create our reality ourselves by making conscious and unconscious decisions (timing of pregnancy, choice of hospital etc.).
- Every woman has the right and the ability to give birth the way it suits her.
- The body of a woman is meant for a natural birth.
- Medical assistance at birth is an interference with natural processes.
- A lot of women lose touch with their bodies and instinctive knowledge and therefore trust textbook authority more than themselves.
- Women can practise using their instinctive knowledge again.
- Women can know instinctively whether things are going well or not and whether their unborn baby is well or not.
- Every birth can be totally different from any other, corresponding to the needs and individuality of mother and child (length of birth, intensity of contractions etc.).
- Home birth is something self-evident and should not need to be fought for.
- All parents should be able to decide for themselves whether home or hospital birth is what they want.
- It is possible to have a beautiful and natural birth experience in hospital, as long as the parents know what they want, what to expect and are able to communicate and assert themselves with the staff of 'their' hospital.

I believe that
- Even in a 'bad' hospital there is a possibility for a good birth experience.

○ It is a tremendous experience for the father to be part of the birth of his child and that this intensifies his relationship to his wife and child.

○ Even if the father missed the birth, or the instant bonding between mother and child could not take place, all is not lost. As long as there is awareness and desire, all this can be made up for.

PARENTHOOD

I believe that

○ Spontaneous mother or father love, seldom 'happens' to be there immediately after birth, but that it grows gradually over hours, days, weeks and months (just as love at first sight is a rare thing amongst adults).

○ It is something very precious and special to feel and look at a newborn child.

○ Newborn children know and feel a lot more than we are able to understand.

○ Most newborn children need body contact and peaceful movement.

○ Some newborn children actually want to have peace and quiet totally by themselves without any stimulation or contact.

○ Newborn children are just as individualistic as adults regarding physical closeness, light, noise, music, bath, sleeping position, eating pattern etc.

○ Many newborn children want the continuous body warmth of their parents and prefer to sleep with them in their bed.

○ Some newborn children prefer to sleep undisturbed on their own.

○ Parents neither suffocate nor spoil their children if they sleep together, if this is what they all want!

I believe that

○ Newborn babies have very individual sleeping patterns and needs.

○ All women could breastfeed.

○ Women who do not want to breastfeed give more to their children when they feed them lovingly with a bottle, than giving them the breast in a resentful way.

○ Some children need a longer and others a shorter breastfeeding period, depending on the individual child and the mother–child relationship.

○ A mother or father who follow the needs of the child completely and at the same time suppress their own needs, do not really serve the child well (as the child will feel the unconscious messages and the double bind).

○ A mother or father who follow their own rules and needs completely and at the same time suppress the needs of the child, do not really serve themelves well (as the child will respond with difficult behaviour or illness).

○ It is possible to find a balance and to respond to one's own needs and at the same time to the needs of the child, especially if the parents learn to trust and deal with their own needs and intuition

Further reading

Antenatal Teaching   Priest, Judy and Schott, Judith, *Leading Antenatal classes*, Butterworth-Heinemann.
Kitzinger, Sheila, *Education and Counselling for Childbirth*, Baillière Tindall
Noble, Elisabeth, *Childbirth with Insight*, Houghton Mifflin, Boston.

Labour Management   Caldeyro-Barcia, R., *Physiological and Psychological Bases for the Modern and Humanised Management of Normal Labour*, Scientific Publication No 858 of the Centro Latino Americano de Perinatologia y Desarolla Humano: Montevideo, Uruguay.
Chard, T. and Richards, M., *Benefits and Hazards of New Obstetrics*, Spastics International Medical Publication.
Cronk, Mary and Flint, Caroline, *Community Midwifery*: A Practical Guide, Heinemann.
Davis, E. *A Guide to Midwifery, Heart and Hands*. Bantam Books.
Flint, Caroline, *Sensitive Midwifery*, Heinemann.
Gaskin, Ina May, *Spiritual Midwifery*, Summertown (available from: The Book Publishing Company, The Farm, 156 Drakes Lane, Summertown, TN 38483, USA).
Inch, Sally, *Birthrights*, Hutchinson.
O'Driscoll, K., and Meagher, D., *Active Management of Labour*, W. B. Saunders Co. Ltd, Philadelphia.

Fetal Development   Nielsson, *A Child is Born*, Faber.
Lux Flanagan, Geraldine, *The First Nine Months of Life*, Heinemann.

Physical Preparation for Birth   Balaskas, Arthur and Janet, *New Life*, Sidgwick & Jackson.
Dale, Barbara and Roeber, Johanna, *Exercises for Childbirth*, Century.

Noble, Elisabeth, *Essential Exercises for the Childbearing Year*, John Murray.

Inkeles, Gordon, *Massage and a Peaceful Pregnancy*, Unwin.

General Books on Pregnancy and Birth

Arms, S., *Immaculate Deception*, Houghton Mifflin, Boston.

Balaskos and Gordon, *The Encyclopaedia of Pregnancy and Birth* Macdonald Orbis.

Beels, Christina, *The Childbirth Book*, Turnstone Books.

Kitzinger, Sheila, *Pregnancy and Childbirth*, Michael Joseph.

Kitzinger, Sheila, *Freedom and Choices in Childbirth*, Viking.

Kitzinger, Sheila, *Giving birth, how it feels*, Victor Gollancz.

Odent, M., *Birth Reborn*, Souvenir Press.

Rose-Neill, Wendy, ed., *The Complete Handbook of Pregnancy*, Sphere.

Stanway A. and P., *Choices in Childbirth*, Pan.

Miscellaneous Aspects of Pregnancy and Birth and Parenthood

Beech, Beverley and Claxton, Ross, *Health Rights Handbook for Maternity Care*, Local Government and Health Rights Project.

Borg, Susan and Lasker, Edith, *When pregnancy fails: coping with miscarriage, stillbirth and infant death*, Routledge & Kegan Paul.

Borg, Susan and Lasker, Edith, *Born too early*, Oxford University Press.

Bradman, Tony, *The Essential Father*, Unwin.

Dalton, Katherine, *Depression after childbirth, how to recognize and treat postnatal illness*, Oxford University Press.

Douglas, Jo and Richman, Naomi, *My Child won't Sleep*, Penguin.

Dunn, Judy, *Sisters and Brothers*, Fontana.

Dunn, Judy and Kendrick, Caro, *Siblings: love, envy and understanding*, Grant McIntyre.

Glover, Barbara and Hudson, Christine, *You and Your Premature Baby*, Sheldon Press.

Hampshire, Susan, *The Maternal Instinct*, Sidgwick & Jackson.

Kitzinger, Sheila, *Experience of Breastfeeding*, Pelican Books.

Kitzinger, Sheila, *Women's experience of Sex*, Dorling Kindersley.

Knight, Bernard, *Sudden Death in Infancy*: *The Cot Death Syndrome*, Faber & Faber.

McKay, S., *Assertive Childbirth*, Prentice-Hall Inc.

Messenger, M., *The Breastfeeding Book*, Century Publishing Co.

Oakley, Ann, *From Here to Maternity – Becoming a Mother*, Pelican Books.

Oakley, Ann, *The Captured Womb*: *History of the Medical Care of Pregnant Women*, Blackwell.

Phillips, Angela, et al., *Your Body, Your Baby, Your Life*, Pandora.

Rank, Maureen, *Free to Grieve*: *Miscarriage and Stillbirth*, Bertary Homes.

Reader, Fran, and Savage, Wendy, *Coping with Caesareans and Other Difficult Births*, Macdonald.

Wakefield, Tom, *Some Mothers I know*: *Living with Handicapped Children*, Routledge & Kegan Paul.

Related Subjects

Benjamin, A., *The Helping Interview*, Houghton Mifflin.
Bond, M., *Stress and Self-awareness*: *A Guide for Nurses*, Heinemann.
Coleman, Vernon, *Bodypower*: *the Secret of Self-Healing*, Thames and Hudson.
Fast, J., *Body Language*, Pan.
Gilmore, S. K., *The Counselor-in-Training*, Prentice-Hall Inc.
Iyengar, *The Art of Yoga*, Unwin.
Kurtz, Ron and Prestera, Hector, *The Body Reveals*: *An Illustrated Guide to the Psychology of the Body*, Harper and Row.
Lineham, Marsha and Egan, Kelly, *Asserting Yourself*, Century Publishing Co.
Lowen, Alexander, *Bioenergetics*, Coventure.
Lowen, Alexander, *Love and Orgasm*, Collier Macmillan.
Maxwell-Hudson, Claire, *The Book of Massage*, Ebury Press.
Melzack, Ronald and Wall, Patrick, *The Challenge of Pain*, Penguin.
Meulenbelt, Anja and Amsberg, Ariana, *For Ourselves*, Sheba Feminist Publications.
Montagu, Ashley, *Touching*: *The Human Significance of the Skin*, Harper and Row.
Murray, Parkes, *Bereavement*, Colin.
Nelson Jones, Richard, *Practical Counselling Skill*, Holt.
Norwood, Robin, *Women who Love too Much*: *When you keep Wishing and Hoping he'll Change*, J. P. Archer, Los Angeles.
Sanders, Deirdre, *Women and Depression*: *a Practical Self-Help Guide*, Sheldon Press.
Stanway, Andrew, *Overcoming Depression*, Hamlyn.
Struna, Monika and Church, Conny, *Self Massage*: *Touch techniques to Relax, Soothe and Stimulate your Body*, Hutchinson.
Thompson & Kahn, *The Group Process as a Helping Technique*, Pergamon.
Whitaker, Agnes, *All in the End is Harvest*: *an Anthology for those who Grieve*, Darton, Longman and Todd.

Books that challenge personal development

Perls, Frederik, *Gestalt Therapy Verbatim*, Bantam.
Mindel, Arnold, *Dreambody*, Routledge & Kegan Paul.
Mindel, Arnold, *Dreambody in Relationship*, Routledge & Kegan Paul.
Leonard, Linda, *Fathers and Daughters*, Shambala Publications.
Leonard, Linda, *On the Way to the Wedding*: *Transforming the Love Relationship*, Shambala Publications.
Perera, Sylvia Brinton, *Descent to the Goddess*, Inner City Books.
Perera, Sylvia Brinton, *The Scapegoat Complex*: *Towards a Mythology of Shadow and Guilt*, Inner City Books.

Whitmont, Edward, C., *Return of the Goddess*: *Femininity, Aggression and the Modern Grail Quest*, Routledge & Kegan Paul.
Miller, Alice, *The Drama of Being a Child*, Virago Press.
Dowling, Colette, *The Cinderella Complex*, Fontana.
Yaloh, Irvin, Do, *Existential Psychotherapy*, Basic Books, New York.

Index